# EMERGENCY HOSPITALS FOR COVID-19

## CONSTRUCTION AND OPERATION MANUAL

Editior-in-Chief
**Yan Zhi**

Translator
**Yan Ge**

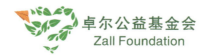

卓尔公益基金会
Zall Foundation

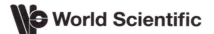

**World Scientific**

NEW JERSEY · LONDON · SINGAPORE · BEIJING · SHANGHAI · HONG KONG · TAIPEI · CHENNAI · TOKYO

*Published by*

World Scientific Publishing Co. Pte. Ltd.

5 Toh Tuck Link, Singapore 596224

*USA office:* 27 Warren Street, Suite 401-402, Hackensack, NJ 07601

*UK office:* 57 Shelton Street, Covent Garden, London WC2H 9HE

**British Library Cataloguing-in-Publication Data**
A catalogue record for this book is available from the British Library.

**EMERGENCY HOSPITALS FOR COVID-19**
**Construction and Operation Manual**

Copyright © Zall Foundation, 2020

ISBN 978-981-122-302-0 (hardcover)
ISBN 978-981-122-303-7 (paperback)
ISBN 978-981-122-304-4 (ebook for institutions)
ISBN 978-981-122-305-1 (ebook for individuals)

To learn more about this book, please visit
**https://www.worldscientific.com/worldscibooks/10.1142/11903**

Desk Editor: Dong Lixi

Typeset by Art Deparment

# EMERGENCY HOSPITALS FOR COVID-19

## CONSTRUCTION AND OPERATION MANUAL

# Contents

## Chapter 4 COVID-19 Emergency Hospitals Operation

## Chapter 5 Emergency Hospitals Logistics Support

# Foreword

The novel coronavirus (SARS-CoV-2) is a newly emerging pathogen, and has the characteristics of strong infectivity and fast propagation. The transmission of SARS-CoV-2 occurs through droplets and can happen through close personal contact with infected persons without effective containment measures. The 2019 coronavirus disease (COVID-19) is an example, and China and other countries have identified and reported a large number of such cases.

Facing the outbreak of the COVID-19 pandemic, with such high patient numbers overwhelming the admission capacities of infectious diseases hospitals, Zall Foundation proposed the construction of COVID-19 Emergency Hospitals in order to effectively respond to the surging number of COVID-19 cases. Emergency hospitals involve the conversion of existing hospitals that currently do not have, or have insufficient admission capacities for infectious disease patients, into emergency hospitals that focus solely on receiving COVID-19 cases. COVID-19 Emergency Hospitals have played an important role in China's epidemic prevention and control by efficiently easing the problems of insufficient ward beds and inadequate admission capacities of infectious diseases hospitals.

Based on the experience of constructing and operating these emergency hospitals in strict adherence to relevant medical standards and regulations, this booklet has been compiled by the Zall

Foundation crew who participated in the rebuilding and supporting of emergency hospitals. It aims to provide useful reference to the reconstruction of existing hospitals and practice of expanding medical resources for all other regions around the world, to effectively contribute to pandemic control.

Yan Zhi

**Founder of Zall Foundation**

April 2020

# Chapter 1

# Background of COVID-19 Emergency Hospitals Construction

## 1.1 Background

Infectious diseases are caused by pathogenic microorganisms; the diseases can be spread, directly or indirectly, from one person to another. Among various types of infectious diseases, the respiratory infectious disease has the highest infection rate, which poses the greatest danger to population health status.

The treatment of infectious diseases should follow stricter requirements for medical environment and protective measurements of treatment and prevention than normal medical institution standards. The patients can be only treated in a professional infectious diseases hospital, in order to prevent further cross-infection between patients and medical staff and to decrease the risks of disease outbreak. With the rapid development of medical technology and improvements in public health management, the epidemic has been contained and brought under full control. This has resulted in the number of professional infectious diseases hospitals being much smaller than normal medical institutions; additionally, the relevant medical supplies and resources would not be sufficient during a disease outbreak. In early 2020, COVID-19 diseases spread rapidly worldwide in a very short time, resulting in inadequate and insufficient medical resources and supplies, which lead to the proposal on the Construction of Emergency Hospitals.

With the COVID-19 outbreak in Wuhan, Hubei, high patient numbers were overwhelming the admission capacities of designated infectious diseases hospitals, which led to insufficient medical supplies fulfilling the treatment needs. In response to the surging number of COVID-19 cases, Zall Foundation proposed the "COVID-19 Emergency Hospital" construction plan. Along with seven professional medical institutions, Zall Foundation suggested converting seven hospitals with no admission capacities for infectious disease patients into emergency hospitals that focus solely on receiving suspected and confirmed COVID-19 patients, which minimize the time and monetary costs. The seven selected hospitals include: The Eighth Hospital of Wuhan, Wuhan Hanyang Hospital, Huanggang Central Hospital Dabie Mountain Regional Medical Center, Wuhan Huangpi People's Hospital Panlongcheng Branch, Luotian No.2 People's Hospital, Jianli People's Hospital and Suizhou Central Hospital. By collaborating with professional medical institutions, among the renovations of Zall 's seven COVID-19 Emergency Hospitals, the shortest hospital renovation took only two days, and the longest took just five days. In total, 4583 wards were provided after renovation, where 2,833 confirmed and suspected patients in Wuhan, Huanggang, Suizhou and Jingzhou etc., were treated and cured.

As mentioned earlier, COVID-19 Emergency Hospitals are established in the context of the epidemic. Hence, the emergency hospitals focus only on the treatment of suspected and confirmed COVID-19 cases. By converting existing professional medical institutions into hospitals focused on COVID-19 patients, it solves the problems of insufficient medical supplies and inadequate admission capacities and plays an important role in providing medical treatment and support.

## 1.2 The Definition of COVID-19 Emergency Hospitals

The basic idea of  COVID-19 Emergency Hospitals is to convert existing hospitals that currently do not have, or have insufficient admission capacities for infectious disease patients, into emergency hospitals that focus solely on receiving suspected and confirmed COVID-19 cases. After the renovation, the treatment environment, equipment and facilities, and operational management of these designated hospitals will have the same standard as a professional infectious disease hospital. The purpose of the establishment of the COVID-19 Emergency Hospitals, is to provide suspected and confirmed patients with medical care and frequent monitoring. The source of infection can also be isolated, leading to a major increase in recovery rate and decrease in infection rate. The reconstruction of existing hospitals involves less time and money, and compensates for the shortcomings of existing hospitals by expanding the admission capacity and medical supplies more effectively.

## 1.3 The Function of COVID-19 Emergency Hospitals

(1) Screening and Triage

The fever clinic should be set up to diagnose patients through the use of laboratory tests, imaging examination and epidemiological investigation. This will help doctors to classify patients into normal patients with fever, suspected patients or confirmed patients. Different medical treatment will be then provided more efficiently.

(2) Isolated Observation and Treatment on Suspected Patients

Before the nucleic acid testing (NAT), all suspected patients from the fever clinic should be observed separately. This will effectively decrease the chance of transmitting the virus to healthy people or being infected by confirmed patients.

## (3) The Admission and Referral of Confirmed Patients

Confirmed patients should be provided with immediate medical treatment in isolated wards. Patients will be discharged once all criteria are met. For severe and critical patients with worsening condition, they should be transferred to designated higher-level hospitals for COVID-19.

# Chapter 2

# COVID-19 Emergency Hospitals Project Design

The design of COVID-19 Emergency Hospitals should strictly comply with relevant regulations and standards. The construction of emergency hospitals project is designed following the principles and guidelines under the Construction Codes on Hospitals for Infectious Diseases Control (GB 50849-2015) and Construction Standards and Regulations on Hospitals for Infectious Diseases Control (Standard 173-2016).

## 2.1 COVID-19 Emergency Hospitals Project Design

(1) The signage system with functions including guidance and management should be implemented in COVID-19 Emergency Hospitals.

(2) All areas in COVID-19 Emergency Hospitals should be barrier-free and accessible.

(3) Hospitals should be strictly divided into restricted areas and isolated areas, with barrier gates placed between these areas. Logistics support facilities and essential living engagement supplies should be placed in restricted areas, whereas receptions, paramedical rooms, wards, ventilation systems, medical waste disposal facilities, temporary morgues, sewage treatment stations and other medical support facilities should be placed in isolated areas. Restricted areas should be located in the upwind direction of isolated areas.

(4) Layout plan should comply with the principle of "three zones and two passages". Three zones are namely: contaminated zone, semi-contaminated zone (potentially contaminated zone) and clean zone.

Clean zone: for medical staff who have low risk of exposure to patients' blood, body fluid, pathogenic microorganisms and other contaminated or infected materials. Confirmed patients with infectious disease are prohibited from entering the area.

Semi-contaminated zone: located between contaminated zone and clean zone, for medical staff who have medium risk of exposure to patients' blood, body fluid, pathogenic microorganisms and other contaminated or infected materials.

Contaminated zone: confirmed and suspected patients with infectious disease are being treated and cured in this area. Blood, body fluid, secretion, medical waste and any contaminated materials should be disposed of in this area.

Furthermore, an operation workflow chart should be clearly informed and explained to all medical staff involved. The design of workflow should be unidirectional from clean zone to contaminated zone. There should be a buffer room between different areas, with wash basins and dirt buckets for polluted medical waste and surgery gowns. This will decrease the risk of cross infection between medical staff.

"Two passages" refer to the health worker passage and patient passage. Cleansing passages and contaminant transferring passages should be strictly separated to avoid any unnecessary interaction between medical staff and patients. The entrance and exit of the health worker passage should be located at the end of the clean zone, while the entrance and exit of the patient passage should be located at the end of the contaminated area.

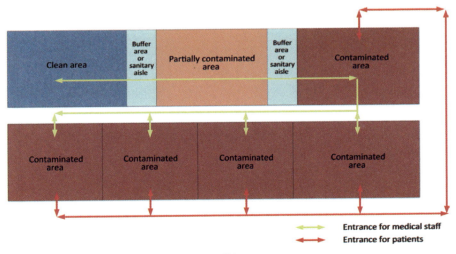

Fig. 2-1 "Three Zones and Two Passages" Design

(5) The layout of the main medical building should allow for the safe, convenient, reasonable and efficient functional linkage between the clinical reception, medical laboratory, inpatient and other main departments which enhance the effectiveness of operation and management.

(6) Interval distance between buildings should satisfy the needs of epidemic prevention and control. The distance between the restricted area and isolated area should be no less than 30m. The distance between buildings inside the isolated area should be no less than 20m.

(7) Complying with the hospital scale, there should be at least two entrances and exits. They should not be adjacent to main streets. The ambulance decontamination site and facilities should be set near the entrance and exit of the ambulance.

(8) The sewage treatment plant should be located on low lying ground. It should have easy access to the urban drainage pipe after strict disinfection procedure.

## 2.2 Reception Area Design

(1) The location should be near the main entrance and exit.

(2) A clear clinical guide for incoming patients should be placed at the entrance to avoid overcrowding and cross infection.

(3) The entrance and exist of admission reception should be placed with buffer rooms.

(4) The consulting rooms, observation rooms, X-ray rooms, ultrasound rooms, electrocardiogram (ECG) rooms, treatment (preparation) rooms, dispensing rooms, temporary contaminant storage rooms, disinfection rooms, sanitary ware rooms, on-call rooms, doctor's offices and toilets for medical staff should be set up.

(5) Patients can only access the consulting rooms, X-ray rooms, ultrasound rooms and ECG rooms with the patient passage under the guidance of medical staff. All other facilities can only be accessed from the medical staff passage.

(6) There should be a patient passage that directly links the admission reception and ward area. This decreases the risk of further disease transmission.

## 2.3 Ward Area Design

(1) The wards with negative pressure and intensive care unit (ICU) should be provided for critical and severe patients, or "super spreaders".

(2) There should be a consulting room and a telemedicine room for second opinion.

(3) Division of inpatient areas should be based on the number of suspected patients, confirmed patients with mild symptoms and severe patients. Suspected patients should be assigned to the single bed ward. Confirmed patients can be assigned to the single bed ward or multi-bed ward. Severe patients, critical patients and "super spreaders" should be treated in the wards with negative pressure or ICU.

(4) Every inpatient area should be complemented with nurse stations, treatment rooms, disposal rooms, doctor's offices, on-call rooms, disinfection rooms, cleansing rooms, personal protective equipment (PPE) storerooms, food preparation rooms and boiler rooms.

## 2.4 Inpatient Room Design

(1) The position of the bed should be parallel with the wall with clear glass. There should be one to two beds in a single ward (one bed is better).

(2) For the ward with multiple beds, the passages between beds should be no less than 1.1m. The distance between the wall and bed should be no less than 0.8m.

(3) The corridor in the single bed ward should be no less than 1.1m.

(4) The toilet in every ward should be complemented with a closet, shower equipment and basins.

(5) The door of the patient room should directly open to the corridor.

(6) The resuscitation room should be near the nursing station.

(7) The width of the patient room should be no less than 1.1m. An observation window should be placed on every door.

(8) Ventilation of the room should be in good condition. Patients can access fresh air outside through the window. Otherwise, an exhaust fan and ventilation system should be installed in the ward.

(9) Rail and anti-collision facilities should be placed on the walls in corridors.

(10) There should be observation windows and delivery windows placed between wards and medical staff corridors. Pass-through chambers should be used on delivery windows.

## 2.5 Medical Laboratory Design

(1) When designing the layout plan, consideration should be given to the separation of patient waiting areas and medical staff diagnosis offices. There should be buffer rooms between medical staff working areas.

(2) Centralised areas of medicine and medical equipment should be located in clean zones, while daily-use medicine and equipment should be allocated in semi-contaminated zones.

## 2.6 Electrical and Intelligent Management Design

(1) Power system in the ward with negative pressure should be isolated and separated from others. Strong and weak electrical circuits and sockets should be properly sealed. Lighting and illumination control in the ward with negative pressure should controllable from both the ward and clean zone.

(2) Electrical circuits in different areas should be separately installed according to the division of clean, semi-contaminated, and contaminated zones. Major electrical installation should be located in the clean zone.

(3) Ceiling lamps in the ward with negative pressure should be properly sealed. During installation, any gap should be properly sealed as well. Materials of lamp shade should not be fragile, but with high transparency. The surface of the shade should be plain and easy to clean and disinfect.

(4) Ultraviolet (UV) sterilizers and germicidal lamps should be installed in clean zone passages, filth cleaning rooms, toilets, inpatient rooms, waiting areas, treatment rooms, wards and operating rooms.

A device should be complemented with UV sterilizer in order to prevent any wrongful action. Switches should be placed at least 1.8m above the ground.

## 2.7 Water Supply and Drainage Design

(1) The draining pipe and ventilation pipe should be separately installed for contaminated zone, semi-contaminated zones and clean zones. Pipes should be made of corrosion-resistant materials.

(2) The valves of the main pipes and branches of water supply should be located in clean or semi-contaminated zones.

(3) All hygiene equipment and floor drain should be complemented with water seals. Water seals should be no less than 50mm. Non-frequently used drains should be properly sealed.

(4) Rainwater of infectious area should be collected in the reservoir and go through a strict disinfection process before being distributed to urban sewerage and drainage pipes.

(5) Contaminated liquid from hospitals should be centrally collected. After disinfection, it should be transferred into a septic tank, then distributed into the liquid disposal station. Contaminated liquid in the disposal station should go through a secondary biochemical process, before being distributed into urban sewerage and drainage pipes.

## 2.8 Ventilation and Air Conditioning Design

(1) Mechanical air supply and air exhaust systems should be installed in the emergency hospitals. Air should be supplied and exhausted through pipes. The systems for different areas should be installed separately for clean zones, semi-contaminated zones and contaminated zones.

(2) The minimum air exchange rate per hour in the negative pressure ward should be 12 times, six times for semi-contaminated and contaminated zones, and three times for clean zones.

(3) The condensed water from air conditioners should be centrally collected. It should first be transferred into the disinfection tank, before being distributed into liquid disposal stations.

(4) In case the air conditioners are used in wards, packaged terminal air conditioners should be able to work independently. If any terminal is discovered to serve two wards simultaneously, the air conditioner should be immediately turned off, and replaced with a variable refrigerant flow (VRF) system.

(5) The negative pressure difference controlled by the exhaust fans and ventilation system should be at the highest in clean zones and lowest in contaminated zones. The pressure difference between isolated wards and corridors should be at least 5Pa. A micromanometer should be installed on the wall of the clean area's corridor walls.

(6) Up-supply and up-exhaust air distribution schemes should be adopted in clean areas and semi-contaminated areas. Up-supply and down exhaust air distribution schemes should be adopted in isolation wards. An air supply outlet should be located on the top of the bed-end, while air exhaust outlet should be located on the top of the head of the bed.

(7) The exhaust fans and ventilation system in the negative pressure ward should be working independently. Filter devices should be complemented with pressure gauges and safety alarms. The ventilation system should not be serving more than six wards simultaneously.

(8) Air supplied to wards should go through low efficiency, medium efficiency, and sub-high efficiency filters in order. Air should go through a high efficiency filter before exhausting. The filter should be placed beside the air exhaust outlet.

(9) The air exhaust outlet in the isolation wards should be placed at least 3m above the ground, away from the supply outlet, doors and entrance for at least 20m in a downwind direction. The location of the

ventilation machine should ensure the negative pressure difference in the ventilation pipes is maintained. The exhaust fans and ventilation system should be controlled in order: Turn on the exhaust fan before the ventilation system; turn off the exhaust fan first and then the ventilation system.

# Chapter 3

# COVID-19 Emergency Hospitals Reconstruction

## 3.1 Reconstruction Procedure

The reconstruction of professional medical institutions into COVID-19 Emergency Hospitals involves steps shown in Fig. 3-1.

(1) Referral of Non-COVID-19 Patients

To avoid the infection of the existing non-COVID-19 inpatients in the hospital, these patients should be transferred to other hospitals or back to home before the reconstruction takes place.

(2) Evaluate the Current Hospital Conditions and Analyze the Reconstruction Procedure

The current situation of the hospital should be evaluated based on the hospital environment, ward area layout, patient room design, water supply, drainage system, etc. The procedure should be further modified and improvised based on the construction standards of Emergency Hospitals for COVID-19.

(3) Reconstruction Project Design

The above evaluation and analysis results should be considered when designing the construction schemes for hospital renovation.

(4) Construction

The preparation of materials and equipment should consider the needs and requirements of the reconstruction process.

(5) Project Delivery and Operation

After the reconstruction, the project should be evaluated and inspected comprehensively. If all relevant criteria and standards are met, the hospital should begin operation and start to receive and treat COVID-19 patients.

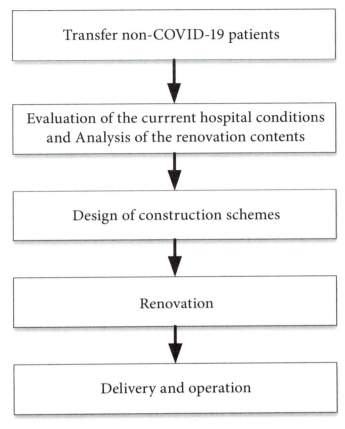

Fig. 3-1 Reconstruction Process of Emergency Hospital for COVID-19

## 3.2 Reconstruction Project Design

The existing hospitals and facilities are partially reconstructed into temporary emergency hospitals for COVID-19 patients in the shortest time. It is the most realistic and accessible way to increase the medical resources and supplies for controlling the epidemic, and to improve the admission capacity for COVID-19 patients. The reconstruction project plan should strictly follow the project design of emergency hospitals in Chapter 2.

## 3.2.1 Reconstruction of Hospitals' Environment

(1) Hospitals should be strictly divided into contaminated zones, semi-contaminated zones and clean zones. An operation workflow chart should be clearly informed and explained to all medical staff involved. There should be a buffer room between different areas, with a separate basket for the contaminated medical and surgery suits.

(2) Medical staff passages and patient passages should be separately designed. Moreover, cleansing passages and contaminants passages should be strictly separated to avoid any unnecessary interaction between medical staff and patients. The entrance and exit of the medical staff passage should be located at the end of the clean zone, while the entrance and exit of the patient passage should be located at the end of the contaminated zone.

(3) Set up a special passage for the prevention and control of infectious diseases in existing hospitals, with prevention containment facilities.

(4) The facilities and vehicles which are not involved in the epidemic prevention and control around the emergency hospitals should be evacuated. For the nearby buildings which are located within 20m

from emergency hospitals, necessary isolation measures should be taken (suspended use if needed). Citizens living in the vicinity should be properly informed by signs and announcements.

(5) Indicate the location for the loading/unloading of medical supplies and equipment, and temporary storage space for epidemic prevention and control purposes.

(6) Indicate the ambulance cleaning and disinfection areas.

(7) Further environmental safety and protection measures should be taken for the medical waste and sewage disposal stations.

## 3.2.2 Reception Area Reconstruction

(1) Set up a fever clinic at the entrance of the hospital.

(2) Overall arrangement to the reception area should stick to the principle of "three zones and two passages".

(3) Mark out the screening area at the outpatient entrance.

(4) Make sure the reception area is provided with the consultation room, observation room, x-ray room, ultrasound room, ECG room, treatment (preparation) room, sewage storage room, disinfection room, tool cleaning room, on-call room, locker room, doctor's office, doctor's washroom, etc.

(5) Patients can only access to the observation room, X-ray room, ultrasound room, and ECG room from the patient passage under the guidance of medical staff. All other facilities can only be accessed and entered from the medical staff passage.

(6) There should be a patient passage that links directly to the admission reception and ward area. This decreases the risk of further disease transmission.

## 3.2.3 Ward Area Reconstruction

(1) Make overall arrangement to the ward area following the principle of "three zones and two passages".

(2) The negative pressure wards and ICU should be provided for critical and severe patients, or "super spreaders".

(3) There should be a consulting room and a telemedicine room for second opinion.

(4) Division of inpatient areas should be based on the number of suspected patients, confirmed patients with mild symptoms and severe patients.

(5) Make sure the working area of each ward is provided with nurse stations, treatment rooms, disposal rooms, doctor's offices, nurse's offices, on-call rooms, disinfection rooms, filth cleaning rooms, bedding and clothing warehouse, diet preparation room for patients, boiler room, etc.

## 3.2.4 Renovation of Normal Isolation Wards

(1) In the multi-bed ward, the distance between two parallel beds should be no less than 1.1m, and the distance between the bed and the wall should be no less than 0.8m.

(2) The corridor in the single bed ward should be no less than 1.1m.

(3) The wards should be equipped with oxygen delivery, suction and other bedside treatment facilities, as well as call and intercom facilities. Make sure that there is enough room at the bedside for X-ray machines, ventilators, etc.

(4) There should be observation windows and delivery windows placed between wards and medical staff passages. Pass-through chambers should be used on delivery windows.

## 3.2.5 Renovation of Negative Pressure Isolation Wards

The procedure to modify normal wards into negative pressure isolation wards is as shown below. See Fig. 3-2.

(1) Each negative pressure ward should be equipped with a toilet. A buffer room should be set between the passage for medical staff and the ward, where an automatic or touchless faucet wash basin is provided. Pass-through chambers should be used on delivery windows.

(2) The air supply and exhaust ventilation system should be prevented from short circuit conditions. The location of the supply outlet should allow the fresh air to first flow through the working area for medical staff, and then to the wards. The air supply outlet should be located on the ceiling. The air outlets of wards, consulting rooms and other contaminated areas should be located on the lower part of the room. The bottom of the air outlet in the room should be no less than 100mm above the ground.

(3) Each negative pressure isolation ward should be equipped with a supply ventilation system with an air volume of 1,500m3/h. The air supplied to wards should go through low efficiency, medium efficiency, and sub-high efficiency filters in order. There should be two exhaust systems, with one equipped with high efficiency filters. The air exhaust should be filtered by the HEPA filter and then discharged.

The HEPA filter for the exhaust should be installed beside the exhaust outlet in the room. Sealed valves should be installed on the air supply and exhaust pipes in each negative pressure isolation ward. The sensor systems are equipped to control the variable frequency fans, to ensure that 5Pa negative pressure is maintained between the negative pressure ward, anteroom and corridor.

(4) The negative pressure isolation ward should be the special first level load. Different low-voltage busbars from the existing substation (distribution room, electrical shaft) provide power to the wards by a two-way power system, with one way for the emergency section, and a pair of power distribution boxes equipped appropriately in the ward for the power supply to the ward ventilation system.

(5) The exhaust fans and ventilation system should be controlled in order.

(6) ELV (extra low voltage) intelligent system

① The existing weak current system (data port, TV port, medical staff intercom port, fire detector, etc.) in the ward remains unchanged.

② A building equipment's monitoring system is implemented to the ward, which automatically controls the ventilation system and monitors the differential pressure in the contaminated and partially contaminated areas.

③ In the ward, an access control system is added to control the passages for medical staff and patients, as well as the transition between contaminated and clean zones in the negative pressure wards.

④ A video monitoring system is implemented to the ward, with two-way voice and video communication functions.

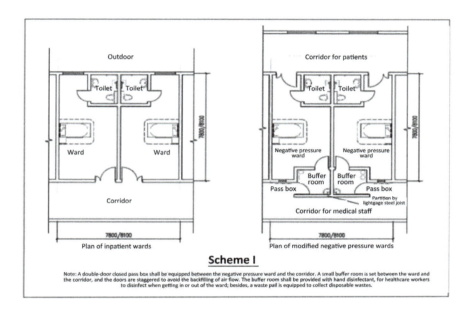

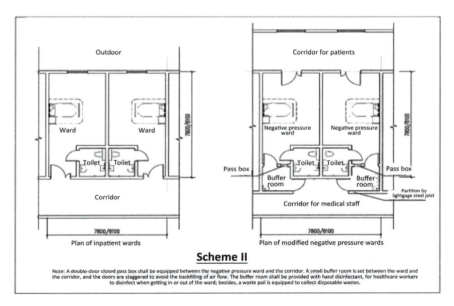

Fig. 3-2 Renovation of Negative Pressure Ward in Emergency Hospital for COVID-19

## 3.2.6 Medical Laboratory Construction

Following the principle of "three zones and two passages", centralized areas of medicine and medical equipment should be located in clean zones, while daily-use medicine and equipment should be allocated in semi-contaminated zones. Consideration should be given to the separation of patients waiting areas and consultation areas. There should be buffer rooms placed between medical staff working areas.

## 3.2.7 Electrical and Intelligent Reconstruction

(1) Power system in the ward with negative pressure should be isolated and separated from others. Strong and weak electrical circuits and sockets should be properly sealed.

(2) The lighting fixtures in negative pressure isolation wards and clean rooms should be cleaned and sealed, and installed on the ceiling.

(3) UV sterilizers and germicidal lamps should be installed in clean zones, toilets, inpatient rooms, waiting areas, treatment rooms, wards and operation rooms.

## 3.2.8 Water Supply and Drainage Reconstruction

(1) The draining pipe and ventilation pipe should be separately installed for contaminated zones, semi-contaminated zones and clean zones.

(2) The valves of main pipes and branches of water supply should be located in clean or semi-contaminated zones.

(3) All hygiene equipment and floor drain should be complemented with water seals. Water seals should be no less than 50mm. Non-frequently used drains should be properly sealed.

(4) Floor drains in the consulting rooms, nurse rooms, treatment rooms, examination rooms, washrooms isolated from the ward, etc. should be closed. There may be floor drains in the washroom of the ward, but regular inspection is required to replenish water for the water seal of floor drains.

(5) Make sure the outdoor sewage discharge inspection wells have closed manhole covers. The drainage pipe network should be equipped with vent stacks, with the vent 2.0m above the ground.

## 3.2.9 HVAC (Heating, Ventilation and Air Conditioning) Reconstruction

(1) Mechanical air supply and air exhaust systems should be installed in the emergency hospitals. Air should be supplied and exhausted through pipes. The systems for different areas should be installed separately for clean zones, semi-contaminated zones and contaminated areas.

(2) The minimum air exchange rate per hour in the negative pressure ward should be 12 times, six times for semi-polluted and polluted areas, and three times for clean areas.

(3) The condensed water from air conditioners should be centrally collected. It should be first transferred into the disinfection tank before being distributed into liquid disposal stations.

(4) In case the air conditioners are used in wards, packaged terminal air conditioners should be able to work independently. If any terminal is discovered to serve two wards simultaneously, the air conditioner should be immediately turned off, and replaced with a VRF system.

(5) Make sure the isolation ward maintains a negative pressure difference of no less than 5Pa with its adjacent and connected buffer room and corridor. A micromanometer should be installed on the wall of the buffer room in the clean area of each isolation ward.

(6) Up-supply and down-exhaust air distribution schemes should be adopted in isolation wards.

(7) Air supplied to wards should go through low efficiency, medium efficiency, and sub-high efficiency filters in order. Air should go through a high efficiency filter before exhausting. The filter should be placed beside the air exhaust outlet.

(8) The air exhaust outlet should be placed at least 3m above the ground, and away from the supply outlet, doors and entrance for at least 20m in a downwind direction. The location of the ventilation machine should ensure the negative pressure difference in the ventilation pipes is maintained.

(9) Make sure the sewage drains and vent pipes in the ward areas are not connected to the drain and vent pipes in the non-ward areas. Good ventilation conditions around the vent pipe orifice of the upper roof should be ensured, and gas disinfection facilities should be provided at the vent pipe orifice if conditions permit.

# 3.3 Reference Cases of COVID-19 Emergency Hospitals for Admission of Diagnosed Patients

For the regions with critical epidemic situations and inadequate medical resources, where the confirmed patients cannot be sufficiently admitted, the renovated emergency hospitals for COVID-19 are solely used to admit the confirmed patients. Taking Zall Changjiang Emergency Hospital (The Eighth Hospital of Wuhan) and Zall Hanjiang Emergency Hospital (Wuhan Hanyang Hospital) as examples, this section introduces the renovation of the COVID-19 Emergency Hospitals for the admission of confirmed patients.

## 3.3.1 Zall Changjiang Emergency Hospital

In order to alleviate the severe shortage of medical resources after the outbreak, Zall Foundation had worked with The Eighth Hospital of Wuhan to reconstruct the North Wing of the hospital. On January 30, 2020, Zall Changjiang Emergency Hospital was officially opened, which is also the first Zall Emergency Hospital for COVID-19. The Hospital has been equipped with a total of 300 beds, mainly for the admission of confirmed COVID-19 patients, and cumulatively treated 560 patients during its operation. The layout plans of the hospital renovation are shown in Fig. 3-3 and Fig. 3-4.

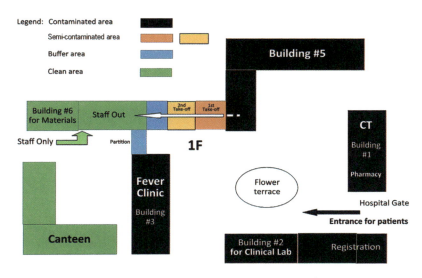

Fig. 3-3 Layout Plan of Zall Changjiang Emergency Hospital 1F

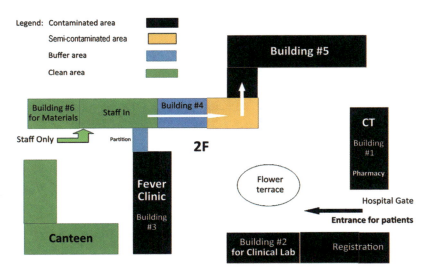

Fig. 3-4 Layout Plan of Zall Changjiang Emergency Hospital 2F

### 3.3.2 Zall Hanjiang Emergency Hospital

On February 1, 2020, Zall Foundation worked together with Wuhan Hanyang Hospital in the renovation of Zall Hanjiang Emergency Hospital, which is solely focused on the confirmed COVID-19 patients. The general inpatient area was transformed into an isolation ward area in line with the standard of "three zones and two passages" within three days. After reconstruction, Zall Hanjiang Emergency Hospital increased its admission capacity to 260 beds and treated a total of 487 patients during its operation. See Fig. 3-5, 3-6 and 3-7 for the renovation of the Hospital.

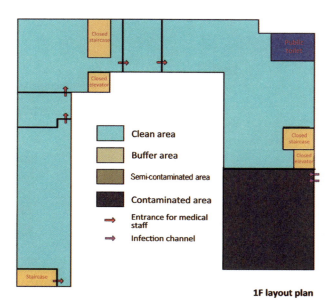

1F layout plan

Fig. 3-5 Construction Plan for Renovation of Internal Medicine Building 1F of Zall Hanjiang Emergency Hospital

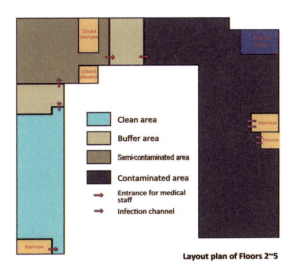

Fig. 3-6 Construction Plan for Renovation of Internal Medicine Building 2-5F of Zall Hanjiang Emergency Hospital

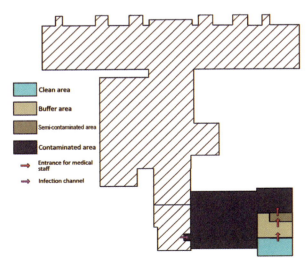

Fig. 3-7 Construction Plan for Paramedical Building of Zall Hanjiang Emergency Hospital

# 3.4 Reference Cases of COVID-19 Emergency Hospitals for Admission of Suspected Patients

For the regions with less critical pandemic conditions but still face inadequate medical resources, where the confirmed patients are fully admitted but the suspected patients cannot be tested and treated, the emergency hospitals are developed mainly used to admit the suspected patients. Taking Zall Panlongcheng Emergency Hospital (Panlongcheng Branch of Huangpi District People's Hospital) and Zall Luotian Emergency Hospital (The Second People's Hospital of Luotian County) as examples, this section introduces the reconstruction project of COVID-19 Emergency Hospitals for the admission of suspected patients.

## 3.4.1 Zall Panlongcheng Emergency Hospital

On February 7, 2020, Zall Foundation and Huangpi District People's Hospital worked together to build the Zall Panlongcheng Emergency Hospital. It involved renovating the inpatient wards of Internal Medicine and Pediatrics in Panlongcheng Branch of Huangpi District People's Hospital into isolation ward areas with the principle of "three zones and two passages" in line with the specification standards, and set up a total of 100 beds, solely used for the admission of suspected COVID-19 patients. During its operation, the hospital treated a total of 358 patients, and 123 patients have been cured. The layout plan of the hospital renovation is shown in Fig. 3-8.

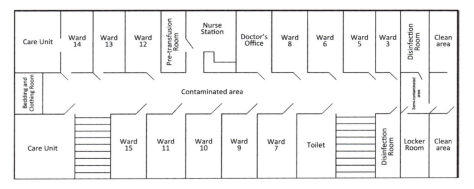

Fig. 3-8 Layout Design for Isolation Wards of Zall Panlongcheng Emergency Hospital

## 3.4.2 Zall Luotian Emergency Hospital

On February 7, 2020, the Second People's Hospital of Luotian County and Zall Foundation jointly set up Zall Luotian Emergency Hospital. The Hospital has set up a total of 100 isolation wards totalling with 500 beds, mainly for the admission of suspected COVID-19 patients, During its operation, 192 patients have been treated and 180 patients have been cured. The layout plans for hospital renovation are shown in Fig. 3-9 and Fig. 3-10.

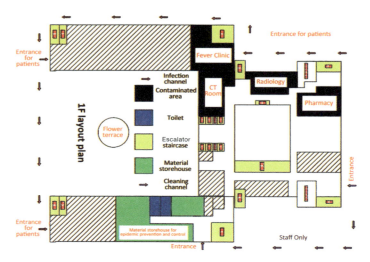

Fig. 3-9 Layout Design of Zall Luotian Emergency Hospital 1F

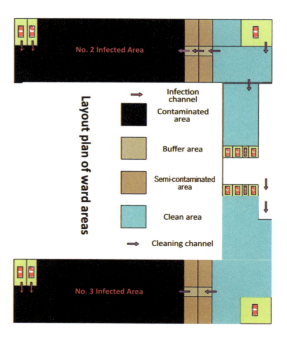

Fig. 3-10 Layout Plan of Ward Area of Zall Luotian Emergency Hospital

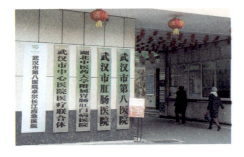

Seven Emergency Hospitals
set up by Zall Successively

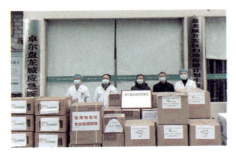

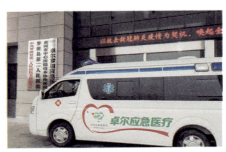

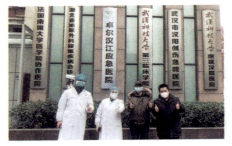

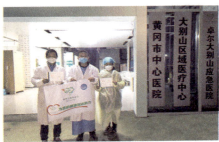

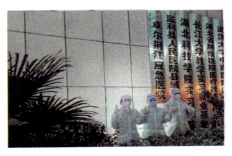

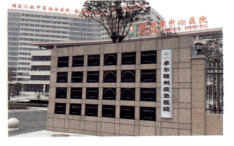

Fig. 3-11 Zall Emergency Hospitals

# Chapter 4

# COVID-19 Emergency Hospitals Operation

## 4.1 Training Program for Medical Staff

### 4.1.1 Training Program Design

The training program will be designed by specialists with extensive experience in teaching and epidemic prevention work from various clinical departments to ensure breadth of knowledge. The design of the program is in strict adherence to relevant medical standards and regulations, which will be tailored according to the actual conditions and situation of the respective hospital. The training courses and assessments mainly cover the procedures relating to proper hand hygiene, donning and doffing procedure of protective masks, gloves, goggles, face shields, protective suits and isolation gowns. Hierarchical protection, pre-examination and triage, as well as diagnosis, treatment and care should also be included.

## 4.1.2 Training for Medical Staff with Standardized Quality

Mentor team members will be selected from doctors and nurses of the clinical skills training center. The training program for mentors consists of three stages. At the end of each stage, all selected mentors will be assigned into different groups, while the group leader is responsible for the evaluation of all trainee mentors, in order to ensure that standardized teaching quality has been delivered by the mentor team.

## 4.1.3 Scientific Design of Training Program

Based on clinical departments, experience level and professional fields, all existing medical staff should be trained in order of expertise. To maximize the training efficiency, the program is divided into two parts: self-learning of theoretical materials and clinical operation training. Participants must complete theoretical self-study before participating in the onsite training. The onsite training procedure includes pre-class tests, watching teaching videos, detailed instructions given by mentors, practical simulation exercises and feedback given from the after-class assessment. During training, medical staff are able to directly apply the skills they have learnt to the practical operation.

### 4.1.4 Multi-Perspectives Evaluation

While the mentor team regularly evaluates the medical staff training performance from feedback collected, staff performance will also reflect the problems and inefficiencies that appear in the training program. Attention also needs to be paid to suggestions and requests from medical trainees, which can be used to improve the teaching quality. See Fig. 4-1.

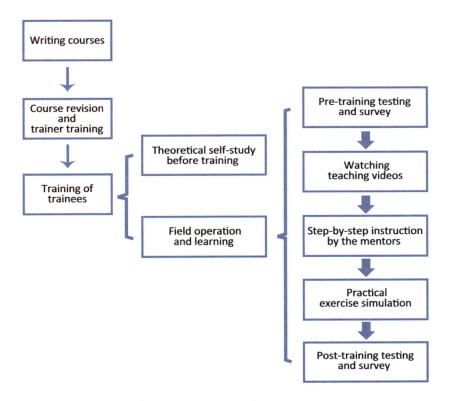

Fig. 4-1 Training Procedure for Medical Staff

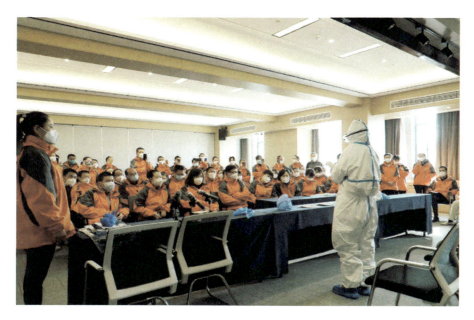

Fig. 4-2 Pre-employment Training for the Medical Team from Xi'an International Medical Center Hospital Invited to Aid Zall Changjiang Emergency Hospital in Wuhan

## 4.2 Patient Admission and Treatment

### 4.2.1 Pre-examination and Triage

The purpose of a scientific method of pre-examination and triage is to comprehensively monitor the condition of all patients, and screen those with high risks of infection. Appropriate treatment in fever clinics in a timely manner will be provided to high-risk patients, which decreases the chance of cross infection. The three-level triage system is shown below:

## (1) Level-1 triage

Pre-examination and triage rooms will be set up for patients with fever in the outpatient department. The infrared temperature thermometer is used to monitor the body temperatures of patients who enter the outpatient department. In the event, a patient with a fever (body temperature > 37.3$^0$) is identified, their temperature should be remeasured with a mercury thermometer immediately. Meanwhile, their epidemiological information will be questioned. If the remeasured temperature is still higher than 37.3$^0$, they must be accompanied by medical staff to the fever clinic for treatment regardless of their epidemiological information.

## (2) Level-2 triage

Temperature monitoring points are set up at every nurse station in the outpatient department in order to monitor the body temperatures of all patients in a timely manner, and screen the patients with fever. Meanwhile, the epidemiological information will be collected from patients with fever. Patients with epidemiological evidence shall be sent to the fever clinic accompanied by a nurse. For patients without epidemiological evidence, they shall be guided to the fever clinic for further examination. After the possibility of COVID-19 infection is ruled out, they will be asked to return to the outpatient department.

(3) Level-3 triage

When diagnosing patients, the outpatient physician should ask them whether they have a fever; if so, enquire about the epidemic medical history. For patients with epidemic history, the outpatient physician shall inform the nurses, who will accompany patients to the fever clinic; for patients without epidemiological evidence, they shall be guided to the fever clinic for further examination. After the possibility of COVID-19 infection is ruled out, they will be asked to return to the outpatient department.

## 4.2.2 Patient Admission Procedure

The physicians will first conduct laboratory inspection, imaging examination and epidemiological investigation to the patients in the fever clinic. The non-suspected patients will be treated and then asked to be quarantined at home for observation, while the suspected patients are provided with treatment in isolated wards, with NAT which will be taken twice, 24 hours apart. If the results are negative, the patients are given general treatment and then asked to be quarantined at home for observation; if the NATs are positive, the patients shall be further evaluated based on the symptoms and examination results. The patients with mild COVID-19 symptoms will be transferred to the Fangcang Shelter Hospital for treatment; the severe patients will be asked to be hospitalized for appropriate treatment in isolation. If patients fulfil the discharge criteria in the later stages, they will be transferred to the "Rehabilitation Station" (the isolation station for patients to receive rehabilitation treatment and medical observation) under quarantine observation and health monitoring for another 14 days.

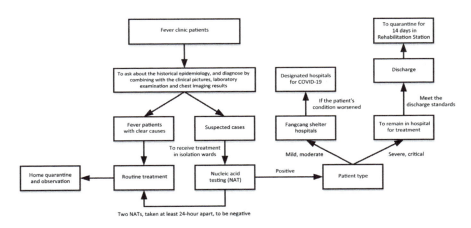

Fig. 4-3 Workflow of Patient Reception/Admission

## 4.2.3 Patient Diagnosis Criteria

(1) Diagnostic criteria for suspected COVID-19 patients

With integrated analysis by combining the epidemiological evidence and clinical symptoms, a patient would be defined as suspected case if one of the following is met: the patient has any of the epidemiological characteristics along with any of two following clinical presentations or the patient has all three clinical presentations if there is no clear historical epidemiology.

① Epidemiological evidences:

(a) History of travel to or residence in an affected area and its surrounding areas, or in other places where cases have been reported within 14 days prior to the morbidity.

(b) In contact with SARS-CoV-2 infector (with positive results for the nucleic acid testing) within 14 days prior to the morbidity.

(c) In contact with patients who have fever or respiratory symptoms from an affected area and its surrounding areas, or from places where cases have been reported within 14 days before the morbidity.

(d) Clustered cases (two or more cases with fever and/or respiratory symptoms in a small area, such as families, offices, schools within two weeks).

② Clinical presentations:

(a) Fever and/or respiratory symptoms;

(b) The imaging characteristics of COVID-19;

(c) Normal or decreased white blood cell (WBC) count, normal or decreased lymphocyte count in the early stage of onset.

If two NATs, taken at least 24 hours apart, of a COVID-19 suspected case are negative, and the SARS-CoV-2 virus specific IgM and IgG antibodies are negative after seven days from onset, the diagnosis of such suspected case can be ruled out.

(2) Diagnostic criteria for confirmed COVID-19 patient

Suspected cases can be diagnosed as confirmed cases if they have one of the following etiological or serological evidence:

① Real-time fluorescent RT-PCR indicates positive for SARS-CoV-2 nucleic acid;

② Viral gene sequence is highly homologous to known SARS-CoV-2;

③ SARS-CoV-2 specific IgM and IgG antibodies are detectable in serum; SARS-CoV-2 specific IgG antibody is detectable in serum or reaches a titration of at least 4-fold increase during convalescence compared with the acute phase.

(3) Clinical classification criteria for confirmed COVID-19 patients

① Mild cases. The clinical presentation and symptoms are mild, and there is no sign of pneumonia on imaging.

② Moderate cases. There are fever and respiratory symptoms, and pneumonia can be found on imaging.

③ Severe cases. Adult cases meeting any of the following criteria:

(a) Shortness of breath, RR ≥ 30 breaths/min;

(b) Oxygen saturation ≤ 93% at rest;

(c) Partial pressure of oxygen (PaO₂)/fraction of inspired oxygen (FiO₂) ≤ 300 mmHg (1 mmHg = 0.133 kPa).

In high altitude areas (altitude > 1000 meters), $PaO_2/FiO_2$ shall be corrected according to the following formula: $PaO_2/FiO_2$*[atmospheric pressure (mmHg)/760].

Cases with chest imaging that shows obvious lesion progression (>50%) within 24 to 48 hours shall be managed as severe cases.

Child cases meeting any of the following criteria:

(a) Shortness of breath (< 2 months old, RR ≥ 60 breaths/min; 2 to 12 months old, RR ≥ 50 breaths/min; 1 to 5 years old, RR ≥ 40 breaths/min; > 5 years old, RR ≥ 30 breaths/min), excluding the effects of fever and crying;

(b) Oxygen saturation ≤ 92% at rest;

(c) Trouble breathing (moaning, nasal fluttering, and infrasternal, supraclavicular and intercostal retraction), cyanosis, and intermittent apnea;

(d) Drowsiness and convulsions;

(e) Refusal of food or difficulty in feeding, and signs of dehydration.

④ Critical cases. Cases meeting any of the following criteria:

(a) Respiratory failure occurs and mechanical ventilation is required;

(b) Shock;

(c) With other organ failure that requires ICU care.

## 4.2.4 Clinical Treatment for Patients

Suspected cases shall receive treatment in isolation in a single ward, confirmed cases can be admitted to the same ward, and critical cases shall be admitted to ICU as soon as possible.

The treatment and medical care provided for patients shall strictly comply with the newly issued COVID-19 Diagnosis and Treatment Program, Nursing Standards for Severe and Critical COVID-19 Patients, and Treatment Guidelines for Severe and Critical COVID-19 Patients.

## 4.2.5 Psychological Intervention Strategy for Patients

With such high patient numbers that are overwhelming the admission capacity, it is possible that patients will also generate negative feelings including depression and more. Hence, an appropriate level of psychological crisis intervention and sufficient mental health consultation for patients is essential in order to make medical treatment more effective.

(1) Confirmed patients
① Newly isolated and treated patients

Patient mentality: numbness, denial, anger, fear, anxiety, depression, disappointment, complaining, insomnia, aggression, etc.

Intervention principles: focus on giving mental support and showing empathy. Treat patients with patience, try to stabilize their emotions and assess the risk of suicide, self-injury, and violent acts in the early stage.

Intervention:

(a) Understanding that these emotional responses from patients are normal responses when facing intensive stress. Be mentally prepared in advance, showing professional care even when facing aggressive and negative acts from patients, for example, not quarrelling with the patient or getting excessively involved.

(b) Given the understanding of the mental status of patients, psychological crisis intervention shall be given in addition to medical treatment, such as assessing the risks of suicide, self-injury and violent acts in a timely manner, providing appropriate mental support, and avoiding having direct conflict with the patient. Patients can consult with a psychiatrist if necessary. Explain the importance of the isolation treatment to patients and encourage patients to build confidence towards future treatment.

(c) Emphasizing the purpose of isolation to the patients, explaining that it is not only for better observation and treatment, but also for the greater benefit of our family and community. Patients should be informed about the key characteristics of the treatment given and the effectiveness of any necessary intervention.

② Patients in isolation and treatment

Patient mentality: In addition to the possible emotional responses mentioned earlier, loneliness and fear of the disease may result in conflict rising with doctors, loss of faith in future treatments, or the opposite, namely unrealistically high expectations for the treatment.

Intervention principle: having direct communication more frequently with patients and providing essential information to stabilize their mental condition. Having consultation with a psychiatrist if necessary.

Intervention:

(a) Based on patients' mental status, objectively and truthfully explain their health conditions, as well as the disease outbreak, so that patients are aware of the current situation.

(b) Encouraging patients to actively communicate with their families. Providing assistance if patients have any reasonable requests.

(c) Encouraging patients to cooperate with doctors in accepting any suggested treatment.

(d) Creating a comfortable environment with a soothing atmosphere that is suitable for patients' recovery.

(e) Having consultation with a psychiatrist if necessary.

③ Patients with respiratory distress, extreme restlessness, and difficulty in expressing themselves

Patient mentality: feelings of imminent death, panic, despair, etc.

Intervention principle: focusing on appeasing and calming the patients, paying attention to emotional communication with them, and helping them build confidence in treatment.

Intervention measures: while calming and appeasing the patient, strengthen the treatment towards the primary cause of mental issues and then relieve the stress.

(2) Patients with fever seeking medical care in the hospital

Patient mentality: panic, restlessness, loneliness, helplessness, being suppressed, depression, pessimism, anger, nervousness, stress of being distanced from others, grievance, shame, disregard for the illness, etc.

Intervention principle: providing basic medicine education and encouraging patients to cooperate with any suggested treatment and adapt to rapidly changing situations.

Intervention:

(a) Assisting patients to understand the true and reliable information and knowledge from authoritative scientific and medical materials.

(b) Encouraging patients to cooperate with doctors in any suggested treatments and with any isolation measures. Ensuring essential living and social engagement needs such as a healthy diet and more.

(c) Helping patients to build up confidence and have faith in future treatments.

(d) Encouraging patients to seek social support to relieve stress by using modern communication methods to contact their friends, family, colleagues, etc.

(e) Encourage patients having consultation with psychologists using assistance hotlines or other online platforms to approach psychological interventions.

(3) Suspected patients

Patient mentality: hoping they do not have the disease, avoiding treatment, fear of being discriminated, or anxiety, asking for excessive treatment, frequent hospital transfer, etc.

Intervention principles: Give timely education and correct

protection. Let patients understand the overall situation and obey instructions. Reduce their pressure.

Intervention:

(a) Receive education on relevant policies, conduct close observation, and seek early treatment.

(b) Adopt necessary protective measures.

(c) Comply with regulations, and report and explain any personal situation according to regulations.

(d) Follow mental health care guidance to relieve stress.

## 4.2.6 Discharge Criteria for Patients

Patients can be discharged if they meet all the following conditions. See Fig. 4-4.

(1) The body temperature has been normal for more than three days;

(2) Respiratory symptoms have improved significantly;

(3) Pulmonary imaging shows a significant decrease of involvement in acute exudative lesions;

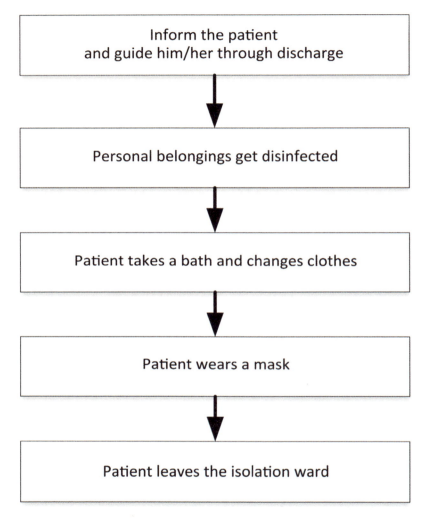

Fig. 4-4 Workflow of Discharge

(4) Nucleic acid tests show negative twice consecutively on respiratory tract samples such as sputum and nasopharyngeal swabs (with sampling interval of at least 24 hours).

After the patient is discharged from the hospital, he/she shall be transferred to the "Rehabilitation Station" to receive the 14-day isolation management. Wear a mask to reduce close contact with others. Strengthen nutritional intake, drink plenty of water (more than 3000 ml per day), and gradually carry out indoor activities. Return to the hospital for follow-up and subsequent visits in two and four weeks after discharge.

## 4.3 Medical Operational Management Policies

### 4.3.1 Management of Fever Clinics

(1) Operation and staffing: Fever clinics shall be opened 24/7 and managed by the emergency department. Trained physicians with clinical experience shall be assigned to screening, consultation, referral, and reporting of suspicious cases. In each fever clinic, there shall be two physicians working simultaneously, with two nurses providing assistance in the clean area. Furthermore, one more nurse shall be deployed in each fever clinic to coordinate work.

(2) Building layout: Divide the building according to the rule of "three zones and two passages" to ensure "unidirectional entry and exit".

(3) Frequent monitoring of ventilation system in the observation room and resuscitation room; if mechanical ventilation is used, the

air flow direction shall be controlled to flow from the clean side to the contaminated side.

(4) Medical staff should be familiar with the epidemiological and clinical characteristics of SARS-CoV-2 infection symptoms, screening suspected patients according to the relevant diagnosis and treatment specifications, take immediate isolation measures for suspected or confirmed patients, and report in a timely manner.

(5) Medical institutions should provide masks for patients and accompanying personnel and guide them to wear the masks correctly.

## 4.3.2 Ward Management

(1) Suspected or confirmed patients should be quarantined immediately and separately; suspected patients should be isolated in single wards, and according to an etiological study, confirmed patients can be placed in the same ward.

(2) Properly implement hand hygiene procedure, and donning/doffing PPE when entering /leaving the isolation ward.

(3) Design procedures for medical staff donning and doffing the PPE; place a flowchart on the door and provide a full-body mirror. There should be staff who are proficient in epidemic prevention and control

work to supervise medical staff on the wearing and taking off PPE to prevent cross infection.

(4) Stethoscopes, thermometers, sphygmomanometers and other medical equipment used for the diagnosis and treatment of suspected or confirmed patients should be used exclusively. If exclusive use of medical equipment cannot be guaranteed, it should be disinfected after use.

(5) Severe patients should be admitted to the ICU or a ward equipped with conditions for monitoring and rescue. No other patients should be admitted to the ICU or the wards equipped with conditions for monitoring and rescue that are meant for admitting severe patients.

(6) Implement a strict patient-visiting system. In principle, no accompanying personnel is allowed. However, if the patient is under special situations, and must be visited, the visitor must strictly comply with relevant regulations and containment measures.

(7) Intensify the ventilation of the ward, and sterilize the air with an air circulating disinfection machine twice per day.

(8)Sheets, quilt covers and pillowcases used by confirmed patients should be contained in double-layer medical waste bags, and the bags should be labeled with "SARS-CoV-2 infection" and sent to the starch washing and disinfection supply center for disinfection; Disinfect pillows, bedding, and mattress pads with a bed unit sterilizer. If there is visible blood or other body fluid contamination, treat it as infectious waste.

(9) General waste of patients with infectious diseases should be treated as medical waste.

(10) Monitor the body temperature and symptoms of medical staff every day. If any medical staff is found to have fever or respiratory symptoms, his/her health condition should be immediately reported to the department of nosocomial infection management.

## 4.3.3 Patient Management

(1) Isolate suspected or confirmed patients in a timely manner, and guide them into the isolation area according to the specified procedure.

(2) Patients should change into hospital gowns before entering the ward area. After patients' personal belongings and the changed clothes are disinfected according to standard procedure, they should be stored in the designated place and kept by the medical institution.

(3) Instruct patients to choose masks correctly and teach them the right procedure of donning the mask, and promote appropriate cough etiquette and hand hygiene.

(4) Strengthen the management of visiting personnel or accompanying personnel.

(5) For isolated patients, in principle, their movements are restricted to the isolation ward, which reduces the frequency of patient movement and ward change. If the patient really needs to leave the isolation ward or area, corresponding measures should be taken, such as wearing a surgical mask, to prevent the patient from causing contamination to other patients and the environment.

(6) When a suspected or confirmed patient is discharged from the hospital or transferred to another hospital, he/she can only leave after changing into clean and sanitized clothes. Medical staff are required to carry out disinfection of all the facilities they have been in contact with.

(7) In case of the death of a suspected or confirmed patient, medical staff should deal with the corpse in a timely manner. The treatment process is as follows: fill the corpse' mouth, nose, ears, anus and other open areas with cotton balls or gauzes that contain 3000 mg/L chlorine disinfectant or 0.5% peroxyacetic acid; wrap the corpse with a double-layer cloth sheet, put it in a double-layer corpse bag, and send it to a designated place for cremation with a special vehicle. Personal items used by the patient during hospitalization can go with the patient or be taken home by his/her family members after disinfection.

## 4.3.4 Setup of ICU Ward Area and Human Resource Management in Nursing

(1) Setup of ward area

The setup of the ICU ward area should be based on local conditions and reasonable layouts. It shall be strictly divided into the contaminated zone, semi-contaminated zone and clean zone. Set up a buffer area between the contaminated area, semi-contaminated area and clean area. Post clear signs in each area to prevent accidental entry. At the same time, set up entrances for medical staff and patients and make sure the two entrances are separate.

(2) Equipment and facilities

① First-aid items and medicines: equip the medical institution with a certain number of ambulances and first-aid medicines, oxygen tanks and supporting devices, ECG monitors, ECG machines, defibrillators, syringe pumps, infusion pumps, supplies for endotracheal intubation, portable vacuum extractors, noninvasive ventilators, hemofiltration apparatuses, extracorporeal membrane oxygenation (ECMO) and other devices.

② Disinfectant equipment: air disinfection machine, disinfection machine, air purifier, watering can, etc.

③ Gas and negative-pressure equipment: prepare a wall oxygen system with sufficient pressure and compressed air.

④ Other facilities: refrigerators, treatment vehicles, wheelchairs, medical carts, etc.

(3)Allocation of nurses and scheduling principles

① Manage the nurses based on the patient-to-nurse ratio of 1:6. The recommended duration for each shift is four hours.

② Nurses should be enriched with ICU professional background, and show professional competence and due care.

③ Nurses should be in good health condition and able to undertake high-intensity work.

### 4.3.5 Transfer of Patients

(1) Transfer requirements

① The on-board medical equipment and facilities (including stretchers) placed in ambulances used to transfer patients, should be used exclusively in the ambulance. The driver's cab should be strictly isolated and separated from the carriage, and a special "contaminated" area for placing protection contaminants should be provided in the ambulance. The additional medical supplies include PPE, sanitizer, disinfectant, etc.

② Medical staff should wear full-sets of working suits, isolation gowns, gloves, medical cabs, and surgery masks. The driver should wear working suits, surgical masks and gloves.

③ After the driver and medical staff transfer the patient infected with SARS-CoV-2, they must change into full-set of PPE in time.

④ Ambulances should be qualified for transferring patients with respiratory infectious diseases. When possible, use ambulances with negative pressure for transferring the patients. During transfer, the ambulance should be kept in a hermetic condition. Disinfect the vehicle after using. When transferring severe patients, the vehicle should be equipped with the necessary life-support equipment to prevent the patient's condition from further deterioration.

⑤ To protect the medical staff and drivers against the virus, the disinfection of vehicles, medical supplies and equipment, and the handling of contaminated items process and procedures should strictly comply with safety standards.

⑥ After the ambulance returns, it needs to be disinfected inside-out before transferring the next patient.

(2) Transfer classification and configuration

The full-time chief resident or the second-line physician on duty determines the transfer level, the personnel to be transferred and the items that need to be prepared based on the patient's pretransfer situation and need for supporting means. According to the required supporting level of organ function, the transfer is classified into five levels: primary, intermediate, advanced, relatively contraindicated and absolutely contraindicated.

① Primary: For patients who only need to use a mask to inhale oxygen, use a low-dose vasopressor \[dopamine < 5μg/(kg·min) or norepinephrine < 0.1μg/(kg·min)\]; The transfer personnel needs to include one doctor and one nurse from the related department.

② Intermediate: For patients who need mechanical ventilation, use a medium-dose vasopressor \[dopamine: 5-10 μg/(kg·min) or norepinephrine: 0.1-0.5 μg/(kg·min)\]; The transfer personnel needs to include one physician from the ICU, one respiratory therapist (RT) and one nurse.

③ Advanced: For patients who need high mechanical ventilation support \[oxygen concentration: 60% to 80%, PEEP: 1012 $cmH_2O$

(1cmH$_2$O ≈ 0.098 kPa)\], use high-dose vasoactive drugs \[dopamine: 10-15 μg/(kg·min) or norepinephrine: 0.5-1.0 μg/(kg·min)\]; Patients should be supported by ECMO; The transfer personnel needs to include one chief resident or second-line doctor from the department, one RT, and one nurse, or the ECMO transfer team.

④ Relatively contraindicated transfer: The patient's vital signs are extremely unstable or the internal environment is extremely disordered, and cardiac arrest will occur at any time and the patient needs to be rescued; The mechanical ventilation support required by the patient is very high (oxygen concentration ≥ 80%, PEEP ≥ 10 cmH20); The patient needs extra large doses of vasoactive drugs \ [dopamine ≥ 15 μg/(kg·min) or norepinephrine ≥ 1 μg/(kg·min)\]; It is suggested to rescue the patient on the spot and transfer the patient after vital signs are slightly stable.

⑤ Absolutely contraindicated transfer: Medical staff are performing cardiopulmonary resuscitation on the patient, and after receiving cardiopulmonary resuscitation, the patient's respiratory status is still unstable under extremely high level of support (SpO2 < 90%, SBP < 90 mmHg).

(3) Transfer process

Wear protections→ drive to the medical institution to pick up the patient → the patient put on a surgical mask → place the patient in the ambulance → transfer the patient to the receiving medical institution → disinfect the vehicle and equipment → transfer the next patient.

(4)Process of donning and doffing protective items

Process of donning protective items: wash or disinfect hands → wear a hat → wear a medical protective mask → wear a working suit → wear an isolation gown → wear gloves.

Process of doffing protective items: take off gloves → wash or disinfect hands → take off the isolation gown → wash or disinfect hands → take off the mask and hat → wash or disinfect hands.

Medical staff and drivers should perform hand hygiene before going off work → shower and change clothes.

(5)Ambulance cleaning and disinfection

① Air: Open windows to ventilate.

② Carriage and object surfaces: Wipe and disinfect with hydrogen peroxide spray or chlorine disinfectant.

## 4.3.6 Protection Provided for Medical Staff

(1) Medical institutions and medical staff shall strengthen the implementation of standard preventive measures, manage the ventilation of the consultation rooms and ward area (patient rooms) well, wear surgical masks/medical protective masks, and wear disposal gloves when necessary.

(2) Take protective measures for droplet isolation, contact isolation and air isolation, and implement the following protective measures under different conditions.

① When in contact with the patient's blood, body fluids, secretions, excretion, vomit and contaminated items: Wear clean gloves, and wash hands after taking off the gloves.

② When medical staff may be splashed by patients' blood, body fluids, secretions, etc.: Wear medical protective masks, goggles and impervious isolation gowns.

③ When performing operations that may generate aerosols for suspected or confirmed patients (such as intubation, non-invasive ventilation, tracheotomy, cardiopulmonary resuscitation, manual ventilation before intubation, bronchoscopy, etc.):

(a) Take air isolation measures;

(b) Wear a medical protective mask and conduct tightness test;

(c) Perform eye protection (for example, wear goggles or a face shield);

(d) Wear body fluid-proof long-sleeved isolation gowns and gloves;

(e) Carry out the operation in a well-ventilated room;

(f) Limit the number of people giving care and support in the room to the minimum needed by the patient.

(3) The PPE used by medical staff should meet the relevant national standards.

(4) Surgical masks, medical protective masks, goggles, isolation gowns and other PPE should be promptly replaced when they are contaminated with patients' blood, body fluids, secretions, etc.

(5) Use PPE correctly, wash hands before wearing gloves, and wash hands with running water immediately after taking off gloves or isolation gowns.

(a) Surgical mask: Surgical masks should be worn correctly in the pre-examination and triage area, fever clinics and the entire hospital. Replace the surgical mask immediately when it is contaminated or wet.

(b) Medical protective mask: In principle, use medical protective masks in areas such as fever clinics, isolated observation wards (rooms), isolation wards (rooms) and isolated ICU (area); when collecting respiratory specimens and performing tracheal intubations, tracheotomy, noninvasive ventilation, sputum suction and other operations that may generate aerosols. A medical protective mask is generally replaced every four hours, and can be replaced at any time when it is contaminated or wet. For other areas and diagnosis and treatment in other areas, in principle, medical protective masks are not used.

(c) Latex examination gloves: Latex examination gloves should be used in the pre-examination and triage area, fever clinics, isolated observation wards/patient rooms, isolation wards/patient rooms and isolated ICUs. Put on and take off the gloves correctly and have the gloves be replaced in time. It is forbidden to leave the diagnosis and treatment area with gloves. Hand hygiene cannot be replaced by wearing gloves.

(d) Alcohol-based hand rub: Medical staff should use it when there is no obvious contaminant on the hands during the diagnosis and treatment. It should be used throughout the hospital. The pre-examination and triage area, fever clinics, isolated observation wards/patient rooms, isolation wards/patient rooms and isolated ICUs must be equipped with the alcohol-based hand rub.

(e) Goggles: Use goggles in areas such as isolated observation wards/patient rooms, isolation wards/patient rooms and isolated ICU/patient rooms, and when collecting respiratory specimens, and performing tracheal intubations, tracheotomy, noninvasive ventilation, sputum suction and other operations that may generate splashes of blood, body fluids and secretions. It is forbidden to leave the above-mentioned area with goggles. If the goggles are reusable, they shall be disinfected before reuse. In principle, goggles are not used in other areas and for diagnosis and treatment in other areas.

(f) Protective masks/protective face shields: Use protective masks/protective face shields for the diagnosis and treatment that may generate splashes of blood, body fluids, secretions, etc. If it is reusable, it shall be disinfected before reuse; If it is for single use, it must not be reused. It is forbidden to leave the above-mentioned area with protective masks/protective face shields.

(g) Isolation gowns: Use isolation gowns in the pre-examination and triage area and fever clinics, and use impermeable disposable isolation gowns in isolated observation wards/patient rooms, isolation wards/patient rooms and isolated ICUs. For other departments or areas, use isolation gowns when in contact with patients. Disposable isolation gowns must not be reused. If the isolation gown is reusable, it shall be disinfected before reuse. It is forbidden to leave the above-mentioned area with isolation gowns.

(h) Protective suits: Use protective suits in isolated observation wards/patient rooms, isolation wards/patient rooms and isolated ICU (area). Protective suits must not be reused. It is forbidden to leave the above-mentioned area with medical protective masks and protective suits. In principle, protective suits are not used in other areas or for diagnosis and treatment in other areas.

### 4.3.7 Procedure of Donning and Doffing PPE

(1) Donning procedure of PPE for medical staff entering the isolation ward area and put on PPE

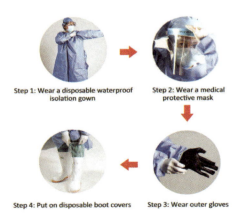

Fig. 4-5 Procedure for Medical Staff Putting on PPE before Entering the Isolation Ward

## (2) Doffing procedure of PPE for medical staff entering the isolation ward area

**(Before returning to the semi-contaminated area from the contaminated area)**

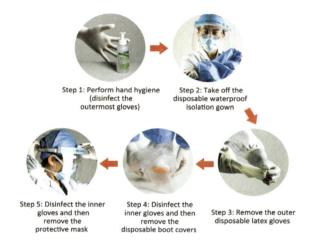

**(Before returning to the clean area from the semi-contaminated area)**

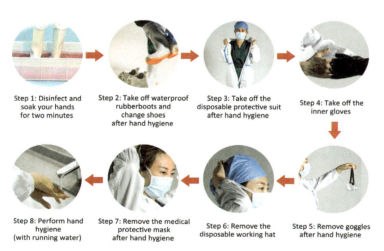

Fig. 4-6 Procedure for Medical Staff Removing PPE before Leaving the Isolation Ward

## (3) Donning and doffing procedure of disposable surgical masks

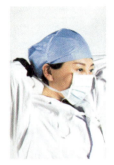 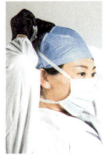 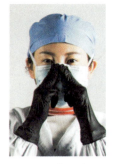 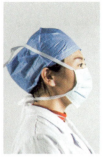

1. The mask must cover the nose, mouth and chin, and the band under the mask shall be tied behind the neck.

2. The upper band of the mask shall be tied to the middle of the head.

3. Put your fingertips on the nose clip. Starting from the middle position, press inwards with your fingers, and gradually move to both sides to shape the nose clip according to the shape of your nose bridge.

4. Adjust the tightness of the mask bands to fit your face.

Fig. 4-7 Donning Procedure of Disposable Surgical Mask

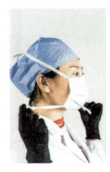 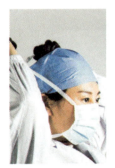 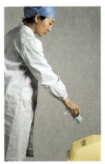 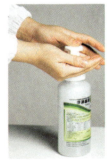

1. First, untie the lower band without touching the front of the mask.

2. Untie the upper band.

3. Pinch the band with your hand and throw it into a medical waste bag.

4. Perform hand hygiene.

Fig. 4-8 Doffing Procedure of Disposable Surgical Mask

## (4) Donning and doffing procedure of N95 respirators

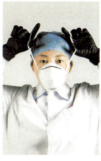 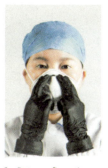 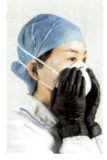 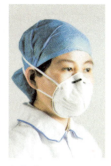

1. The protective mask must cover the nose, mouth and chin, and the tip of the nose clip shall be close to the face. Pull the elastic band of the mask with both hands. Pull it up and over the top of the head, and put it behind the neck and in the middle of the head.

2. Put your fingertips on the metal nose clip. Starting from the middle position, press the nose clip inward with your fingers, and move and press it to the side to shape it according to the shape of your nose bridge.

3. Press the front of the mask with both hands and perform a positive pressure tightness test: Deeply exhale. If it is positive pressure, then there is no air leakage; If there is air leakage, adjust the mask position or tighten the band.

4. Perform negative pressure tightness test: Inhale deeply. If there is no air leakage, the mask will be close to the face. If there is air leakage, adjust the mask position or tighten the band.

Fig. 4-9 Donning Procedure of Medical Protective Mask

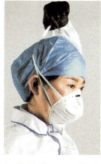 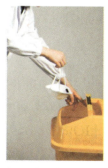 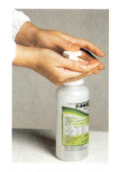

1. Hold the two elastic bands with both hands at the same time, and lift them up and over the head to take the mask off.

2. Pinch the elastic bands with both hands and throw the mask into a medical waste bag.

3. Perform hand hygiene.

Fig. 4-10 Doffing Procedure of Medical Protective Mask

## (5) Donning and doffing procedure of isolation gown

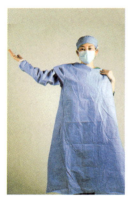
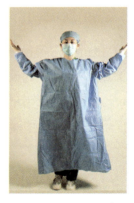
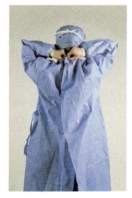

1. Hold the collar with your left hand and put your right hand into the sleeve. Use your left hand to pull the collar upwards to let your right hand be exposed to the air.

2. Now change sides. Hold the collar with your right hand and put your left hand into the sleeve. Let your right hand be exposed to the air. Do not touch your face.

3. Hold the collar with both hands, and fasten the neckband backwards from the center of the collar and along the edge.

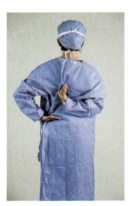
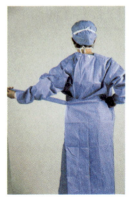
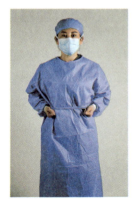

4. Align the hem with your hands behind your back.

5. Fold to one side, hold the fold with one hand, and pull the belt to the fold at the back with the other hand.

6. Cross the ends of the belt behind, go back to the front, and fasten the ends of the belt.

Fig. 4-11 Donning Procedure of Isolation Gown

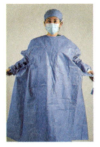
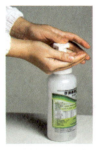
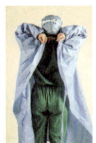

1. Untie the belt and tie a slip knot in front.

2. Disinfect your hands.

3. Untie the band behind the neck.

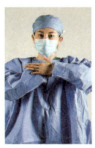
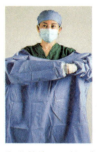
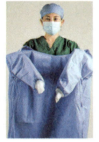

4. Put your right hand into your left sleeve and pull the sleeve off your left hand.

5. Hold the outside of the right sleeve of the isolation gown with your left hand, which is covered by the left sleeve, and pull down the right sleeve.

6. Withdraw your hands gradually from the sleeves and take off your isolation gown.

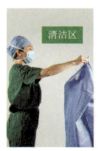
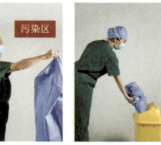

7. Hold the collar with your left hand, and align the two sides of the isolation gown with your right hand. If you hang it in the contaminated area, the contaminated side of the isolation gown faces outwards. If you hand it outside the contaminated area, the contaminated side of the isolation gown faces inwards.

8. When it is no longer in use, roll the used isolation gown into the shape of a package with its contaminated side facing inwards and throw it to the designated recycling place.

Fig. 4-12 Doffing Procedure of Isolation Gown

## (6) Donning and doffing procedure of protective suit

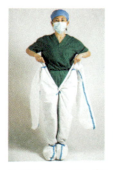 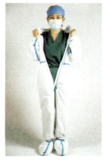 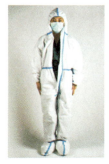 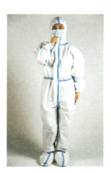

1. First, put on the bottom.
2. Then put on the upper clothes.
3. Put on the hat.
4. Zip up.

Fig. 4-13 Donning Procedure of Protective Suit

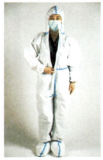 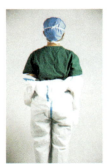 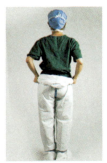 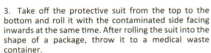

1. Zip up from the top to the bottom.
2. Take off the sleeves.
3. Take off the protective suit from the top to the bottom and roll it with the contaminated side facing inwards at the same time. After rolling the suit into the shape of a package, throw it to a medical waste container.

Fig. 4-14 Doffing Procedure of Protective Suit

## (7) Donning and doffing procedure of goggles or protective masks

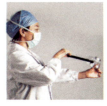 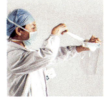 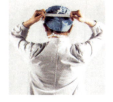 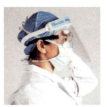

1.  Check for any damage and slack.

2. Grasp the ear or head band of the goggles or protective mask and adjust it to make yourself comfortable.

Fig. 4-15 Donning Procedure of Googles or a Protective Mask

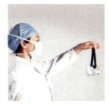 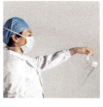 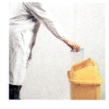 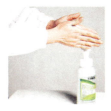

1.  Grasp the end of the ear band of the goggles or the head band of a protective mask, and take off the goggles.

2.  For reusable goggles, place them in a covered container for centralized cleaning and disinfection. For non-reusable goggles, throw them into a yellow medical waste trash can, and then perform hand hygiene.

Fig. 4-16 Process of Taking off Goggles or Protective Clothing Mask

### 4.3.8 Protective Supply Allocation

(1) Zoning based on exposure risk level

According to different exposure risk levels, medical staff who have resumed daily diagnosis and treatment will take on different personal protective measures.

① High-risk exposure areas: All medical staff who directly or may come into contact with patients or their contaminants and the surfaces of the contaminated items and environment. The following departments are included: the ICU, emergency, the pre-examination and triage, fever clinics, emergency surgery, clinical laboratory, delivery room, catheter room, dialysis room and other departments in which invasive operations are performed.

② Low-risk exposure areas: Personnel who are less likely to directly come into contact with patients or their contaminants and the surfaces of the contaminated items and environment. The following areas are included: general outpatient clinics, inpatient wards, medical laboratories, areas for the frontline managing staff and workers (cleaning staff, rotating warehouse staff, security staff, cafeteria staff, mortuary staff, medical waste disposal staff, accompanying staff, etc.).

(2) Allocation standard

In principle, allocate different medical protective supplies according to different risk exposure levels and different job requirements.

① High-risk exposure areas

Items: medical protective suits, medical protective masks, goggles or protective masks, isolation gowns, disposable surgical mask, disposable working hats, disposable medical gloves.

Allocation standard: In the ICU, emergency surgery, clinical laboratory, delivery room, catheter room, dialysis room and other departments in which invasive operations are performed, medical staff must be equipped with medical protective suits, medical protective masks, goggles or protective masks, disposable working hats, and disposable medical gloves when diagnosing and treating all patients who are admitted by emergency department and haven't completed the COVID-19 screening.

② Low-risk exposure areas

Items: Medical protective masks or surgical masks, disposable working caps, disposable medical gloves, working suits or isolation gowns.

Allocation standard: All personnel in the medical institutions should be equipped with these items.

# Chapter 5

# Emergency Hospitals Logistics Support

## 5.1 Material Storage and Support

### 5.1.1 Storage of Common Supplies

(1) Common medicine

As of today, there is no known proven medicine or cure for COVID-19, however, the following drugs can mitigate the disease empirically:

① Alpha-interferon: 5 million unit or equivalent dose each time for adults, adding 2ml of sterilized water, atomization inhalation twice daily.

② Lopinavir / Ritonavir: 200 mg/50mg per pill for adults, two pills each time, twice daily, no longer than 10 days.

③ Ribavirin: suggested to be used jointly with interferon or lopinavir/

ritonavir, 500 mg each time for adults, two or three intravenous injections daily, no longer than 10 days.

④ Abidol: 200 mg three times a day for adults, no longer than 10 days.

⑤ Chloroquine phosphate: 500 mg twice a day for adults, no longer than 10 days.

Apart from the drugs mentioned above, drugs such as antiviral drugs, antibacterial agents, analgesic antipyretic, antitussive, antiasthmatic and expectorant medicine, gastrointestinal drugs, intestinal microecological modulators and immunomodulators can also mitigate the disease. The hospital should reserve sufficient supplies of drugs according to its admission capacity.

(2) Common device and equipment

Testing and monitoring equipment: infrared thermometer, polymerase chain reaction (PCR) detector, patient monitor.

Therapeutic equipment: ventilator, oxygen machine, defibrillators, injection pump.

Disinfection equipment: temperature measurement and sterilization station, UV disinfection lamp [MOU2].

(3) Common protective equipment

Operating caps, surgical masks, N95 respirators, working gowns, disposable coveralls, high-grade protective suits, full-face respirator masks, positive pressure headgears, goggles, disposable isolation gowns, protective shoe covers, disinfectant, etc.

## 5.1.2 Procurement and Supply

The hospital is responsible for tabulating the list of necessary drugs, protective equipment, and devices required, which will be subsequently purchased by the charity institutions. Other than ensuring common medical supplies mentioned in the earlier section, the hospital should also focus on ensuring an adequate supply of drugs related to COVID-19 treatment. The purchase must be made from pharmaceutical companies with legal qualifications. The qualifications of relevant companies and business personnel must be recorded alongside the purchase for transparency and accountability. When there is a shortage of supplies, the hospital should actively negotiate and communicate with the providers, encouraging them to expand the supply chain or transfer the supplies from other regions. Meanwhile, if the purchasing process is difficult, the hospital should actively seek alternative supplies and materials.

### 5.1.3 Donation of Drug and Medicine

The donated drugs and medicines must meet the following requirements and criteria:

(1) For those produced within China, the drug must be a product approved by the local drug regulatory authority, with a valid approval number, and meet quality standards. The validity period must be more than six months before the expiration.

(2) For those produced outside of China, the drug should be approved by the local drug regulatory authority, accepted by international pharmacopoeia, legally produced and listed in the country of registration, and meet quality standards. The validity period must be more than six months before the expiration. If the drug's approval is valid less than 12 months, the drug should be used six months before the expiration date.

## 5.2 Warehouse and Logistics Support

To improve the efficiency of management and resource utilization, the medical and living materials and supplies are under unified management and storage systems. Meanwhile, a professional transport team is formed to allocate supplies in time according to the actual demand.

## 5.2.1 Warehouse Management System

(1) Responsibilities:

① Goods receiving, warehouse entry, returning, storage and protection.

② Loading and unloading, transportation and packaging of supplies.

③ Disposal of waste.

(2) Management Requirements:

① For each arriving shipment of supplies, before the supplies are stored into the warehouse, the go-down entry should be issued once the supplies are checked.

② According to the demand of supplies, after the consignor and the transportation vehicle have been checked correctly, the outbound order is made and signed by the consignor.

③ On a daily basis, the warehouse must make inventory tables and distribution charts for unallocated supplies, and keep the supplies classified and preserved properly.

## 5.2.2 Transportation Management System

Transportation agencies must follow a unified command and coordination plan. They must propose and formulate plausible transportation plans, and deliver the supplies and materials to COVID-19 Emergency Hospital in a safe and timely manner.

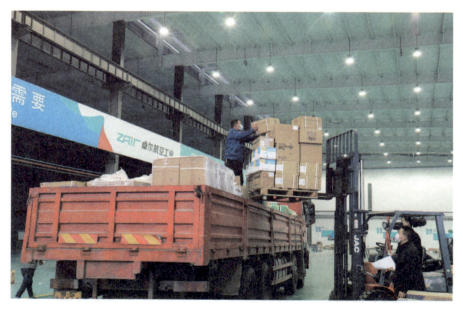

Fig. 5-1 Warehouse of Zall Emergency Hospital

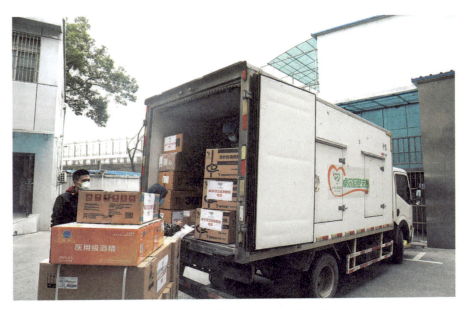

Fig. 5-2 Allocation of Materials of Zall Emergency Hospital

## 5.3 Dietary Nutrition Support

### 5.3.1 Dietary Guidelines

(1) Diet Plan for Patients with mild symptoms and recovery patients

① In order to maintain adequate daily energy, patients should ensure sufficient nutritional intake, such as: daily intake of 250-400g cereal and tubers, which includes: rice, flour, grains and others; daily intake of 150-200g protein, which includes: lean meat, fish, shrimps, eggs, beans and more; consume one egg daily if it is possible, along with 300g of milk and dairy products (yogurt can be selected as it can provide essential probiotics). Moreover, it is important to ensure fatty-acid intake through various types of vegetable oil, especially through those with unsaturated fatty acid. Total fat should reach 25% to 30% of total energy intake.

② Patients should be encouraged to eat more fresh fruits and vegetables: 500g daily vegetables intake and 200-350g daily fruits intake (dark green vegetables would be recommended).

③ Patients should drink enough water (1500-2000ml daily). Patients should drink boiled water or tea. Soup made from vegetables, fish or chicken is also recommended to be consumed before or after meals. Drinking water in small amounts, but more frequently can help increase water intake.

④ Eating wild animals is strictly prohibited. Food with spicy flavor is not recommended.

⑤ A special diet plan will be provided to patients with anorexia and chronic diseases, and elderly patients, with nutrient-intensifying supplements including: proteins, Vitamins A, B, C, D and other types of micronutrients.

(2) Diet Plan for Severe Patients

It is common that severe patients often have decreasing appetite, which leads to insufficient energy and nutritional intake. This will lessen their resistance to the disease. Hence, greater attention should be paid to the dietary plan for severe patients. The following principles should be followed when setting their daily nutritional intake:

① Consuming smaller meals, but more frequently will help increase food intake. Consume liquid food six to seven times a day (liquid diet is easier to swallow and digest). Patients are encouraged to eat more eggs, beans, milk and dairy products, fruit juice, vegetable juice and rice flour. Good protein is also important for daily nutrition intake. During the recovery period, a semi-liquid diet can be taken. When their health condition is stable, a normal diet plan can be provided for patients.

② If food consumed by severe patients fails to meet daily nutrition intake standards, special medical-use food can be provided such as food containing enteral nutritional supplement, under the guidance of medical staff.

③ Under the circumstances of insufficient enteral nutrition, loss of intake ability, or facing a patient with severe gastrointestinal dysfunction, parenteral nutrition should be used in order to maintain basic nutrition daily intake. Parenteral nutrition should be 60% to 80% of total nutritional intake in the early stage, and increased to the full amount when patients' health condition is better.

④ Diet for severe patients should be planned based on body condition, intake and output volume, hepatorenal function and the glucose and lipid metabolism condition of the patients.

(3) Diet Plan for frontline medical support staff

By following the principle of a balanced diet, the diet plan for front-line medial and support staff should comply with the following:

① In order to ensure adequate daily energy intake, male staff are encouraged to consume 2400-2700 kcals a day, while female staff are encouraged to consume 2100-2300 kcals a day.
② Staff should ensure there is daily consumption of protein, such as eggs, milk, meat, fish and shrimps, beans and more.

③ Food with light texture is recommended, and try to avoid eating greasy food. Natural spices can be used as ingredients to increase appetite.

④ Food with enriched vitamins B and C, minerals and dietary fiber is encouraged, along with rice and noodles, vegetables and fruits. Vegetables and fruits such as grapes, spinach, celery, purple cabbage, carrot, tomatoes, oranges, apples and kiwi fruits, as well as homonemeae vegetables such as mushrooms, wood ears and seaweed are recommended for their daily diet.

⑤ Water intake should be 1500ml to 2000ml per day.

⑥ When a normal diet plan cannot meet the daily nutritional intake standard, enteral nutrition supplements can be used under the guidance of medical staff, together with powdered milk and other supplements. Additional 400kcals to 600kcals of oral nutrition supplements should be administered a day, in order to ensure daily energy intake.

⑦ Eating alone should be promoted, to effectively decrease the risk of cross infection during meal times by avoiding gathering.

⑧ Departments which are responsible for diet plans should reasonably adjust measures in line with the conditions of the frontline medical and support staff.

## 5.3.2 Logistics and Distribution Management

The emergency hospitals' own logistics support teams have faced difficulties in delivering sufficient amounts of food for patients and medical staff since the COVID-19 outbreak. Meanwhile, the F&B industry is deeply affected by the epidemic, causing the closing down of restaurants. Faced with such pressing conditions, charities and nonprofit organizations should collaborate with medical institutions, not only for the setting of diet plans, but also for finding suitable logistics and distribution companies to deliver essential food supplies. Taking Zall Hanjiang Emergency Hospital as an example, the logistics and distribution company delivers food to the quarantine building with refrigerated trucks, the hospital's logistics support crew then arranges for staff to pick up the food supplies, then deliver them to different clean areas according to the amount reported. Finally, food will be sent to wards by the nurses on duty.

## 5.4 Hygiene and Disinfection

### 5.4.1 Air Disinfection

Daily basis: At least four times a day. Disinfect the room immediately after suspected or confirmed patients are treated.

Occupied room: (1) Natural ventilation 30 minutes every time. (2) UV air disinfection two hours every time.

Empty room: (1) The disinfection method for "occupied room" is applicable. (2) Disinfection by lamp irradiation.

Final disinfection: Disinfectants such as peracetic acid, chlorine dioxide, hydrogen peroxide, etc. can be used for disinfection by using the ultra low volume spray method. After the disinfection, the room must be ventilated thoroughly.

## 5.4.2 Surface and Environment Disinfection

Disinfection on daily basis: Four times every day

Disinfection on timely basis: After treating suspected or confirmed patients, the room and transfer devices must be disinfected.

Final disinfection: After daily work

Disinfection method: Wipe or spray the object surface with 1000mg/L chlorine-containing disinfectant. After 30 minutes, wipe the surface with clean water. Clean the floor with 1000mg/L chlorine-containing disinfectant, the duration of disinfection must be at least 30 minutes.

## 5.4.3 Floor and Wall Disinfection

Evenly spray and disinfect the surfaces of corridors, lavatories, toilets, waste disposal, medical waste storage rooms and other spaces with 1000mg/L chlorine-containing disinfectant. The process must be at least 30 minutes each time and four times every day. Clean the floor with a 1000mg/L chlorine-containing disinfectant, and the duration of disinfection must be at least 30 minutes, four times every day.

## 5.4.4 Medical Equipment Disinfection

Disposable medical instruments and equipment should be used as much as possible, and the medical waste should be disposed after use. For reusable medical instruments and equipment, first soak them in 2000mg /L chlorine-containing disinfectant for 30 minutes, and then seal in a special container with labeled "COVID-19" for recycling. For disinfection supply centers, pressure steam sterilization is recommended. For devices that are not heat resistant, chemical disinfectant or low-temperature sterilization is preferred.

## 5.4.5 Disposal of Patients' Blood, Excretion, Secretion, Vomit

(1) A small amount of contaminants can be carefully removed by disposable absorbent materials (such as gauze and cleaning cloth) after dipping 5000-10000mg/L chlorine-containing disinfectant, or removed by disinfectant wipes/dry wipes with strong disinfection effect.

(2) A large amount of contaminants should be completely covered with disinfectant powder or bleaching powder containing water-absorbing components. Or they should be completely covered with disposable water absorbing materials before applying sufficient 5000~10000mg/L chlorine-containing disinfectant on the water absorbing materials for more than 30 minutes. They can also be removed by disinfectant wipes/dry wipes with strong disinfection

effect. These contaminants should be carefully removed. Contact with contaminants should be avoided during removal. The contaminants should be treated as medical wastes in concentration. Patients' excretion, secretion and vomits should be collected in a special container and soaked in 20000mg/L chlorine-containing disinfectant with the substance to medicine ratio of 1:2 for two hours.

(3) After the removal and disposal of the contaminant, the surface of the environment and objects should be disinfected. The container holding contaminants should be immersed in 5000mg / L chlorine-containing disinfectant for 30 minutes.

### 5.4.6 Miscellaneous

(1) Patients' cutlery, leftovers and vegetable residue should be disinfected.

(2) During morning care, change the sheets with disposable bed covers. Each bed should have one bed cover. The patients' clothes, sheets, duvet covers and pillowcases should be replaced immediately after contaminated. The bedside table, bed, chair and stool should be wiped and disinfected with disinfectant on a daily basis. After the discharge or death of the patient, the bed cover of the patient must go through a final disinfection.

(3) When collecting patients' clothing, quilts and other textiles, aerosols should be avoided. It is recommended to incinerate them as medical wastes in concentration. Textiles that need to be reused should be soaked in 20000mg/L chlorine-containing disinfectant for 30 minutes before routine cleaning. They should be collected in water-soluble packing bags as infectious textiles and delivered to a cleaning company for cleaning and disinfection. Expensive clothes can be disinfected by ethylene oxide.

## 5.5 Medical Waste Management

### 5.5.1 Classification and Collection of Medical Waste

(1) Define the range of classified collection. Waste produced by medical institutions or hospitals during the treatment of confirmed or suspected patients with COVID-19, including medical waste and household garbage, should be collected, classified and disposed in the same way as medical waste.

(2) Establish strict standards for packaging and containers. Warning signs must be attached to the surface of special packaging bags and sharps containers for medical waste. Before disposing medical waste, careful inspection should be carried out to ensure the container is not damaged or leaking. Foot operated and covered barrels are preferred for waste collection. When the medical waste reaches 3/4 of

the packaging bag or sharps container, it should be sealed effectively and tightly. Double-layer packaging bags should be used to contain medical waste, and gooseneck-type seals should be used for layered sealing.

(3) Collect waste safely. According to the type of medical waste, collect the waste in a timely manner, ensuring the safety of personnel and minimizing the risk of infection. When the surface of the packaging bag and sharps container is contaminated with infectious waste, a layer of packaging bag should be added. It is strictly forbidden to squeeze the bag when collecting disposable clothing, protective clothing and other items after use. Each packaging bag and sharps container should be attached with a label. The label should include the name of medical unit, department, date and type of waste, and marked specifically with "COVID-19".

(4) Process the waste from different zones. For medical waste produced by confirmed or suspected patients with COVID-19 at the fever clinic and wards before leaving the contaminated area, the surface of the packaging bag should be sprayed uniformly and disinfected with 1000mg / L of chlorine-containing disinfectant, or a layer of medical waste packaging bag should be added on the outside. The medical waste generated in the clean zone should be disposed of according to conventional medical waste.

(5) Handle pathogen samples carefully. High-risk waste such as pathogen-containing specimens and related preservation solutions in medical waste should be steamed or chemically sterilized at the place of production, then collected and disposed of the waste in the same way as infectious medical waste.

## 5.5.2 Transportation and Collection of Medical Waste

(1) Management of safe transportation. Before transporting medical waste, the personnel should check whether the label and the seal of the bag or sharps container meet the requirements. While transporting the waste, the personnel should prevent damage to the packaging bags and sharps containers containing medical waste, avoid direct contact with medical waste, and avoid leakage and spread of medical waste. Clean and disinfect the transportation tools with 1000mg / L of chlorine-containing disinfectant after the daily transportation. When the transportation tool is contaminated with infectious medical waste, it should be disinfected immediately.

(2) Management of handover and storage. The temporary storage place for medical waste should be tightly closed and attended by hospital staff, to prevent irrelevant personnel from coming into contact with medical waste. Medical waste should be stored in a separate and temporary area, and handed over to the medical waste disposal unit for disposal as soon as possible. The floor of temporary storage places must be disinfected with 1000mg / L of chlorine-containing

disinfectant twice a day. The medical department, transport personnel, temporary storage staff, and medical waste disposal unit transfer personnel should check and register while handing over the waste, and explain to each other that it originates from patients with pneumonia or suspected patients infected with the new coronavirus so that extra caution can be taken.

### 5.5.3 Disposal of Medical Waste

Irrelevant articles and personal necessities should not be placed or stored in incineration sites. During the incineration, the medical wastes should be properly packaged; After incineration, relevant equipment, containers and sites should be thoroughly cleaned and sterilized. Medical waste disposal equipment should be cleaned and sterilized before repair and maintenance. Sewage generated during the disposal of medical waste (including disinfection and cleaning of delivery vehicles, containers, temporary storage facilities, and disposal of sewage on the ground) should be discharged after being disinfected by centralized sewage treatment facilities.

## 5.6 Mental Health Care and Support

Healthcare workers often face heavy mental and physiological stress caused by the risky and highly intensive work, which may affect their work enthusiasm and performance. With such high patient volume that overwhelmed the admission capacity, it is possible that health workers will be prone to suffer from negative feelings including depression, etc. Hence, it is essential to establish mental health care policies and show our support for frontline healthcare workers.

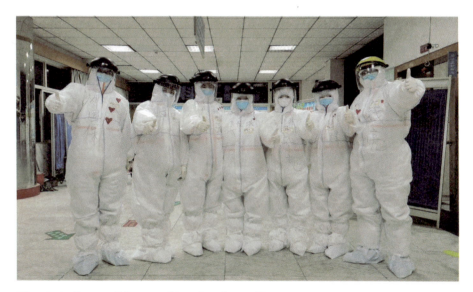

Fig. 5-3 Group Photo of Medical Staff

## 5.6.1 Mental Health Care for Medical Staff

(1) Improving working and leisure facilities

Ensure privacy by providing additional facilities such as single resting rooms for medical staff. Moreover, attention should be paid to the leisure and isolation needs, as well as essential living and social engagements of healthcare workers.

## (2) Work and leisure balance

While providing medical treatment to patients, sufficient rest hours should be provided to medical staff, according to the current epidemic prevention and control conditions, and relevant scientific research. Generally speaking, medical staff should not work consecutively over a month. Frontline medical staff should have a shorter consecutive working period. Deferred holiday leave should be arranged for those who are unable to take leave during the prevention and control working period, after they have completed their mission.

## (3) Enhancing health care facilities for medical staff

Ensure sufficient medical supplies for containment, especially for staff working on the front line. Physical examination should be given to frontline staff, including CT scans and more, which will decrease the risk of cross infection. If any medical staff is found infected, immediate isolation and treatment should be provided.

## (4) Psychological crisis intervention and mental health care consultation

A psychological consulting team should be established which consists of psychologists and other medical staff. Its major responsibility is to assess the health condition of every medical staff, while providing essential guidance. An appropriate level of psychological crisis intervention provided to medical staff and their families is also important, in order to effectively relieve the pressure they face. For medical staff having stress disorder symptoms, more mental intervention should be given, along with rearrangements of their working schedules to ensure adequate down time.

(5) Providing essential care to frontline staff

Understanding the needs and demands of frontline staff and their families, and fulfil reasonable requests from them in a timely manner.

(6) Human resource preferential policies

Based on the evaluation of medical staff's performance in epidemic prevention and control, additional credit should be given to outstanding medical staff. Preferential policies should be adopted by the medical institution's recruitment team; priority should be given to medical staff with outstanding performance in terms of promotion, title evaluation, etc.

(7) Welfare policies

Increasing salary and providing subsidies.

(8) Improving working conditions and ensuring safety at work

Strengthen safety measures and improve working conditions. No tolerance will be given to any direct or indirect discrimination to the medical staff and their families. Legal action will be taken towards tort, intentionally spreading of diseases and disorderly acts.

(9) Strengthen advocacy measures

Give credit and commendation to medical staff who made significant contribution in the epidemic prevention and control and showed outstanding performance.

## 5.6.2 Mental Health Care for Patients

(1) Psychological crisis intervention and mental health care consultation

A psychological consulting team should be established by psychologists and other medical staff. The major responsibility is to assess the health condition of every patient, while providing essential guidance. An appropriate level of psychological crisis intervention provided to patients is also important, in order to effectively relieve their pressure.

(2) Welfare and subsidies policies

Subsidies should be granted for patients with financial difficulties, thus encouraging them to hold positive attitude and cooperate with treatment.

# References

[1]  Ministry of Housing and Urban-Rural Development of the People's Republic of China. GB50849-2014. Architectural Design Code for Infectious Diseases Hospital [S]. Beijing: China Planning Press, 2015.

[2]  Ministry of Housing and Urban-Rural Development of the People's Republic of China. National Development and Reform Commission. Construction Standards 173-2016. Construction Standard for Infectious Diseases Hospital [S]. Beijing: China Planning Press, 2016.

[3]  China Association for Engineering Construction Standardization. The Design Standard of Infectious Diseases Emergency Medical Facilities for COVID-19 [S]. Beijing: China Building Industry Press, 2020.

[4]  Housing and Urban-Rural Development Department of Zhejiang Province. Health and Family Planning Commission of Zhejiang Province. Architectural Design Code for Infectious Diseases Area (Department) of Zhejiang Province [S]. Hangzhou: Zhejiang Standard Design Station, 2006.

[5]  Housing and Urban-Rural Development Department of Zhejiang Province. Technical Guide for Construction of Respiratory Infectious Diseases Emergency Hospital in Zhejiang Province (Trail) [Z]. 2020.

[6]  Housing and Urban-Rural Development Department of Zhejiang Province. Technical Guide for Emergency Renovation of Deadly Infectious Diseases Area (Department) of Zhejiang Hospitals (Trail) [Z]. 2020.

[7]  National Health Commission of the People's Republic of China. Ministry of Housing and Urban-Rural Development of the People's Republic of China. Notice on Issuing Design Guide for COVID-19 Emergency Facility (Trail) [EB/OL]. http://www.gov. cn/zhengce/zhengceku/2020-02/11/content5477301.htm.

[8]  West China Hospital, Sichuan University. Medical Panel for COVID-19 Pneumonia of Sichuan Province. Emergency Prevention Guide for COVID-19 Pneumonia Medical Institution. Chengdu, Sichuan Science and Technology Press, 2020.

[9]  State Council of the People's Republic of China. Notice on Conducting Proper and Precise Prevention and Control of COVID-19 Epidemic According to Law. [EB/OL]. http://www.nhcgov.cn/jkj/ s3577/202002/69b3fdcbb61f499ba50a25cdfld5374e.shtml.

[10] Lv Zhanxiu, Zhou Xianzhi, et al. Management of Modern Infectious Diseases Hospital. Beijing: People's Military Medical Press, 2010.

[11] Huanggang, Lou Tianzheng, et al. Handbook of COVID-19 Prevention and Treatment for Hospital at Community Level [M]. Hangzhou: Zhejiang University Press.

[12] National Health Commission of the People's Republic of China Dietary and Nutritional Guide for COVID-19 Prevention and Treatment [EB/OL]. http://www.nhc.gov.cn/xcs/yqfk dt202002/a69fd36d54514c5a9a34456l88cbc428.shtml.

[13] Hu Bijie, Liu Ronghui, et al. Diagram for SIFIC Hospital Infection Prevention and Control [M]. Shanghai: Shanghai Science and Technology Press, 2015.

[14] National Health Commission of the People's Republic of China Intervention Guide for Emergency Psychological Crisis Caused by COVID-19 Epidemic [EB/OL]. http://www.nhc.gov.cn/j/s3577202001/6adc08b966594253b2b791be5c3b9467.shtml.

[15] Hubei Province Health Committee, Hubei Provincial Department of Education, Hubei Provincial Department of Finance, Hubei Resources and Social Security Department of Hubei Province. Measures on Strengthening Care and Incentives for Healthcare Workers on the Front Line of COVID-19 Prevention and Control [EB/OL]. http://www.hubeigov.cn//zfwj/ezbf/202002/t202002182103386.shtml.

# Acknowledgments

Jack Ma Foundation

Alibaba Foundation

The Eighth Hospital of Wuhan

Wuhan Hanyang Hospital

Huanggang Central Hospital

Panlongcheng Branch of Huangpi District People's Hospital

The Second People's Hospital of Luotian County

People's Hospital of Jianli County

Suizhou Central Hospital

Zall Foundation is a public welfare organization established in Wuhan, Hubei Province, China. Founded by Yan Zhi, Chairman of Zall Holdings Company Limited, the foundation mainly focuses on public welfare activities such as disaster relief, poverty alleviation, student assistance, culture and sport events, and ecological and environmental protection.

After the outbreak of the novel coronavirus disease in 2020, Zall Foundation greatly relieved the pressure of the medical system in Hubei by quickly launching various assistance. They donated a large number of urgently needed medical protection equipment to Hubei for fighting against epidemic; provided materials to renovate existing hospitals into emergency hospitals to treat suspected and confirmed COVID-19 patients; converted public venues to Fangcang Shelter Hospitals to treat patients with mild to moderate symptoms of COVID-19; and offered logistic support to guarantee the smooth operation of these hospitals.

In addition, Zall Foundation actively participates in global fight against COVID-19 by donating medical supplies to 16 countries. It continues to share its experiences by publishing the timely books, *Fangcang Shelter Hospitals for COVID-19: Construction and Operation Manual*, and *Emergency Hospitals for COVID-19: Construction and Operation Manual*. Currently, these two booklets have been translated into more than 20 languages.

---

**Emergency Hospitals for COVID-19: Construction and Operation Manual**

---

Editor-in-Chief: Yan Zhi
Editors: Zhang Liang, Du Shuwei, Tian Xudong, Niu Yadong, Xiong Xiaochuan
Translator: Yan Ge
English Proofreader: Wang Sida
Layout designer: Huang Xuan, Song Jie, Ye Qinyun, Hu Yangfu
Photographer: Fan Ruiqi